And We Write: Surviving Cancer

Let the Healing Begin

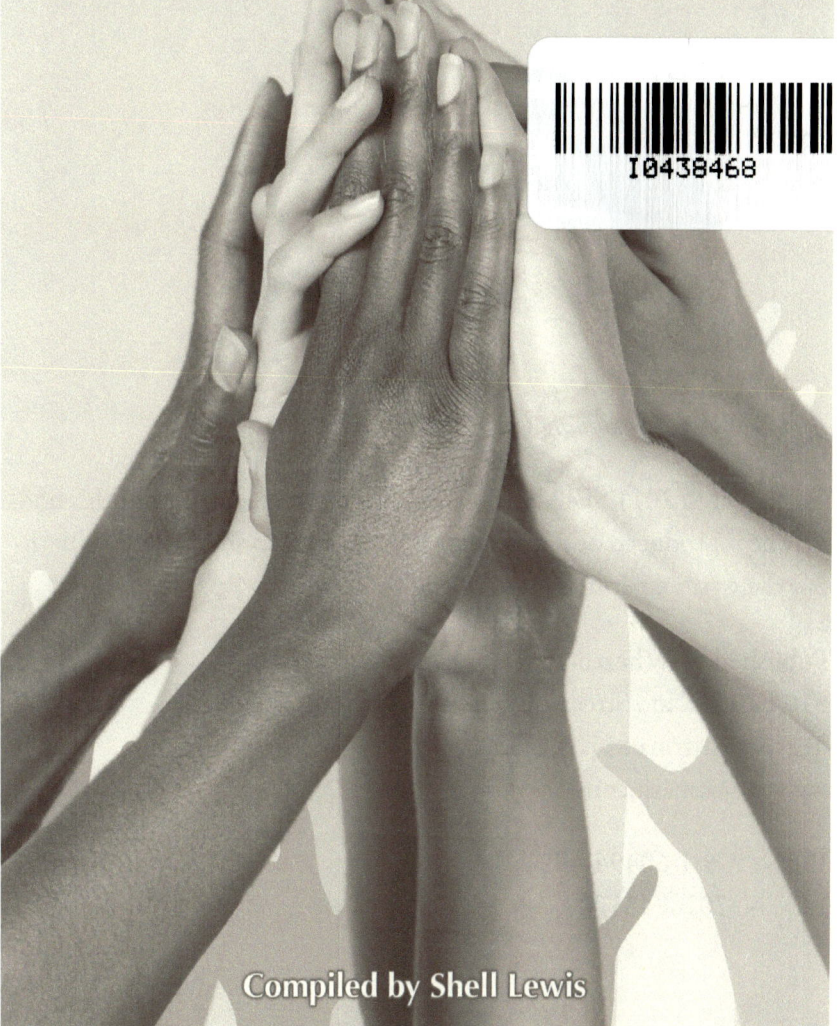

Compiled by Shell Lewis

And We Write: Surviving Cancer; Let the Healing Begin

Published by Wheatmark®
610 East Delano Street, Suite 104
Tucson, Arizona 85705 U.S.A.
www.wheatmark.com

ISBN: 978-1-60494-492-1
LCCN: 2010943170

Let the Healing Begin

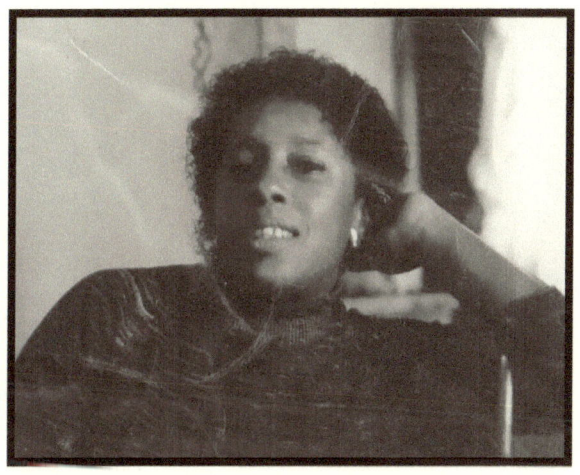

In Loving Memory of Clara May Lewis

They have slithered into my life yet again.
This is just as much for you, Melody,
as it is for you, Mommy.

Contents

Contents

Introduction

My sister and I wanted to find a way to honor our mother, who succumbed to colon cancer on March 29, 2006. How do you provide a fitting tribute? Cancer doesn't just attack an individual; it attacks the individual and his or her loved ones. Both my sister and I knew just how devastated we were by our loss. We also knew that our entire family felt the enormity of our mother's absence. She was truly the backbone of the immediate family. Mom, however, was not egotistic. She was the epitome of selflessness, and I knew that she would want us to include the words of all those who are combating those cancerous, invasive little bloodsuckers that slither into one's body as readily as they slither into everyone's lives.

Quite frankly, I think that I am better understood on paper. I can articulate my thoughts in writing far better than I can verbally. By the time I have finished writing, my jumbled and disjointed thoughts seem a bit more concrete and coherent than when spoken out loud, so I wanted to write. I wanted to create this compilation, providing myself an outlet in which I could sort out my thoughts, thus affording my family the chance to make sense of what we had all experienced and to honor our mother, Mrs. Clara May Lewis, while extending the same opportunity to others.

While I was writing my own entries, I wrote from a place of pain and endurance—that place where words take on new meaning. My ability to write was fueled by some unseen force, some being that seemed to force-feed me words with the ease with which a blind man maneuvers a familiar dwelling.

I believe that all of the entries on the following pages are written from a similar place. Whether that place is in the comedic relief of "Better Boobs" or "Tub Thumping," the testimony and plea made in "My Name Is Prasenjit Chandra," or in the heartfelt, poetic prose of "October Ruse" and "Cancer," the results are all the same. There is meaning in this compilation.

Not everyone will enjoy what the following pages will reveal, but hopefully everyone will have arrived at a sense of peace that will be exclusively their own; somewhere between the lines they will have arrived at their own meaning.

Since my mother's passing, the word mother has become so much more than caregiver, more than the backbone of the family, and more than an ATM, a cook, a cleaning woman, and a hairdresser.

We didn't know what was wrong with Mother.

We were in the dark.

Nothing was known, only an obvious fatigue and loss of weight. Then there was blood. Then there was more blood. Then there was a doctor's visit. Then there was cancer. Even then my father refused to believe it. He was under the impression that she would merely bounce back with that energetic sprightliness to which we had all grown accustomed, but somehow I knew that things weren't as they seemed. This wasn't going to be the comeback for all ages. She was sick—really sick. Even she knew it, but she had this way about her, you know?

As she awaited the results, an uncharacteristically frail woman sat before me, yet her swagger still remained. It was the pride that I was accustomed to seeing on Sunday mornings when we had to get dolled up for church, Bible study, and Sunday school, the pride that went into refashioning every worn ensemble, the pride that made her scold us when we begged, the pride that made her discipline us when we misbehaved, the pride that made her console us afterward, the pride and faith that made her say, "Oh, you are right, you cannot heal me, but somebody else can."

She somehow possessed the ability to turn every unpleasant situation into a celebration for the blessing that was about to come, and we couldn't help but fall in line.

Even after her first surgery—the one during which the tumor was removed along with a portion of her infected ovaries—she emerged unscathed with a sense of renewed devotion to God and a rejuvenated spirit, but I still noticed that she was just a bit winded, just a bit slower than before.

I remember going on vacation. It was a Caribbean cruise with a high school friend. Both my mother and father greeted me upon my return, picking me up from LaGuardia Airport. I was so happy to see her. I still lived at home and was a definite "momma's girl." Just a week away from her seemed like a month; now, in her absence, it feels like an eternity!

A few months prior to my departure, she had surgery, a very invasive procedure to remove a golf-ball-sized tumor from her colon. Her recovery was quick and impressive; nevertheless, the cancer had spread, and no later had I returned had a new growth emerged on her inside right knee. It had materialized in one week. She had developed liposarcoma, a tumor developing in the fatty tissue around her knee.

There is definitely more to my story, which you will read momentarily. First you must embark on your own personal journey. I hope that you enjoy where it takes you and that you will not mind the emotional hurdles that you will encounter along the way. More so, I pray that what you will read will take you on a rewarding and enlightening path on which you'll get a panoramic view of the people and experiences that have touched our lives in various ways, and that we can together put a stop to this disease.

Better Boobs
by Mark Barkawitz

"How do you like my new boob, Mike?" Kelly asked as I approached her on the front porch of her Sierra Madre cottage. She smiled and stuck her left one forward for me to inspect. It was impossible to detect any difference under her sweater and bra.

"Looks good to me." I smiled back. I'm a painting contractor, mostly residential, so I tend to work with a lot of women in their homes. I drink a lot of coffee and tend to talk a lot too, about a lot of things. Sometimes they confide in me. Last year, just as I was putting the finishing touches on Kelly's kitchen remodel, she was diagnosed with breast cancer. Her sister had died a few years ago of the same cancer. Kelly had gone through a lot in the year since I'd seen her: mastectomy, chemo, radiation, recovery, and finally, her new boob. We hugged.

"You look good, kid," I told her.

"Thanks. I feel good." She smiled again. "Gary likes it, too." Gary was her husband.

I laughed. I do that a lot, too.

"So what do you want painted this time?"

"Follow me." I did. I checked out some dry rot in the fascias around the outside of the house and garage and advised her that those boards should be changed instead of repaired.

"Can you do that, too?" she asked.

"Sure." We went inside.

She poured me a cup of coffee. I leaned against the counter and sipped her strong, hot brew, and we gabbed for the next hour or so about her kids and my kids and who was going to what school and playing what sport and whether I was coaching again next season and my wife's new teaching job and the new puppy that Kelly was getting next week and just about everything except cancer. We finally got around to scheduling a start date. I put my empty coffee cup in her sink.

"I have to leave you now."

"You have another job to go to today?" she asked.

"Yup. Or I'd let you feed me, too." She was a good cook. We both laughed. Kelly did that a lot, too. It was probably why we got along so well.

"Next time," she said.

We hugged goodbye, and I hurried out to my truck where I'd left my cell phone on the seat. There was one missed call. I recognized the number: it was Waters, my next job. I called back.

"Haylo?" It was the housekeeper's voice.

"Mariela?"

"Sí. Is that you, Mikey?"

"Sí."

"Mar-rgo wants to know if you still coming today?" Margo Waters was the homeowner. It had been a few months since I'd last worked at the Waters' castle, as I called it. It was an old, two-and-a-half-story, twenty-eight-room, concrete-walled, multimillion-dollar mansion on Pasadena's west side above the arroyo overlooking the Rose Bowl. A home like that was constantly in need of maintenance. It was a handyman's dream, especially because Mr. Waters was an investment banker whose work quite often took him to the East Coast for long spells. I'd painted one room seven years ago and had worked there doing odd jobs on and off ever since.

"I'm on my way. Did you miss me?"

"Oh, sí. You so nice. You always help me."

2

I carried groceries up the back stairs for her, nothing any gentleman wouldn't do for a lady. No big deal.

"I have sooprise," she said.

"For me?"

"No, ees not for you. But ees sooprise."

A few minutes later, I turned into the long driveway that led to the castle. Mariela's was the only car parked in the paved lot on the south side of the estate. I parked next to her SUV, away from the gigantic twin evergreens, one of which leaned over the lot, allowing squirrels to drop half-eaten pine cones from the upper branches—like hand grenades—onto the hoods of unsuspecting guests' parked cars. I opened the tailgate, placed my toolbox on it for easy access—I pretty much worked out of the back of my truck—grabbed a few hand tools I knew I'd need, and headed up the back stairway. Through the row of kitchen windows on the landing, I saw Mariela inside at the sink. I knocked on the door, but opened it myself.

"Morning."

"Hi, Mikey. Coffee ees in microwave for you." She continued to wash dishes in the sink. "Margo go to gym. Leave note for you." Without turning towards me, she indicated with a nod that the note was on the kitchen island.

I turned on the microwave and checked the note. I recognized Margo's handwriting:

-fix latch on cab in butler's pantry

-paint walls in guest room

"Margo's sister went home?"

"Sí."

"How is she?"

Mariela shook her head. "Ees no good. Berry sick."

I nodded. Margo's sister was currently going through what Kelly had gone through last year. But her sister had been pregnant at the time that

3

the cancer was discovered, which had delayed and complicated her treatment, and the cancer had spread. The microwave dinged. I took the cup out, sipped the steamy coffee, and went back to the list:

-replace all burnt-out light bulbs

-move potted trees from east patio to west patio

-assemble automatic cat box

"Automatic cat box?"

"Sí. Mar-rgo get a new kitty."

"Really?" In all the time I'd worked in the castle, the Waters had never had a pet. From under the island, a black paw reached out for my shoelace. I put down the cup, got down on one knee, and bent low. Yellow-green almond-shaped eyes stared back at me from the jet black face of a young feline—too old to be a kitten, too young to be a cat—perched like a sphinx, ready to pounce.

"Hey, there." I reached down to pet its head between ears that were pointed upright. "What's its name?"

"Hair-rball."

"Hairball? That's funny. How you doing, Hairball?" It purred gently. Then I noticed each nail on its front paws was coated with some kind of clear, plastic sheath. I took its paw in my hand to inspect it more closely. "What the heck?"

Still at the sink, Mariela looked down. "Ees so kitty won't scratch furniture."

"You're kidding." I ran my fingers across the floor in front of Hairball, who reached out to stroke my hand with its paw. The soft acrylic sheaths kept its fingernails from digging into the skin on the back of my hand. I had to laugh. "What will they think of next?" Then I remembered the list— "*-assemble automatic cat box*"—and figured I'd find out soon enough.

"How's you knee?" Mariela asked.

"Not bad. Rehab took awhile, but I'm back up to five or six miles a run now." I'd hurt it last summer. I didn't know how; I just woke up one

4

morning and out of nowhere the darn thing was swollen like a volley-ball, wobbly as a loose pipefitting, too. I sipped the coffee and found the loose latch in the adjoining pantry, took the Phillips screwdriver from my back pocket, and carefully tightened the guilty loose screws. "How's your back?" I asked through the doorway.

"Oh, ees bueno. I'm so glad. I tell Mar-rgo ees no more heavy lifting." She had been wearing a brace because of a lower back strain, but it was hard to tell under her baggy sweatshirt if she was still wearing it. I had given her some exercises to try. She dried her hands on the dishtowel and turned to me with a funny, conspiratorial sort of look on her face. "You remember what we talk about last time you are here?"

I thought back.

"Come on." She prodded me. "You remember." She smiled and winked.

"Oh." I did suddenly remember—breast implants. Mariela had lost thirty pounds over the last year and a half but had confessed to being un-happy with how the weight loss had left her breasts, so she had consulted a plastic surgeon in the San Fernando Valley. I glanced down slightly, but the loose-fitting sweatshirt hid any clear indication. So, risking a faux pas, I was compelled to ask uneasily, "Did you do it?"

She pursed her lips and nodded.

"Really?" I looked again more closely. "Obviously you didn't opt for the Ds." Her husband's suggestion as I remembered.

"No." She shook her head. "Ees a full C."

"Ahh. A full C."

"You want to see?"

"What?"

"Come on. I show you." She walked ahead of me, farther into the house. I followed—what else could I do?—through the dining room, where the luminous faces of Renaissance men and women stared judg-mentally down at me from a wall-sized painting, into a small hallway, where she closed the doors at both ends. She turned to me and pulled up the baggy sweatshirt, under which firm twin mounds—like cantaloupe halves—were wrapped snuggly by a cotton crop top.

"Oh." I couldn't help staring, but I didn't figure it was rude in this instance anyway.

"Ees no bra," she stated proudly.

"No bra? You're kidding?"

She shook her head. "No. Ees too sensitive." She covered them up and smiled again. "Eh?"

"To quote my favorite sitcom, 'They're spectacular.' Good for you. Good for your husband, too," I kidded.

"Oh, he crazy now. He keep asking doctor, 'How soon? How soon?'"

"So you haven't tried them out yet?"

"No, no, no." She wagged her index finger like a mother playfully instructing a child.

"Ees too sensitive. Doctor say ees okay for Saturday night."

"Really?" I smiled, thinking of her husband. "This Saturday?"

She nodded and wagged her finger at me again. "Doan you tell no one. Ees secret. No want Mar-rgo to know. I tell her I have back surgery. Take two weeks off. Thees morning she look over while I cook. But I no tell her."

"Yeah, she might get pissed off now that her housekeeper has better boobs." We both laughed.

A door closed with a thud from the kitchen end of the house.

"Ees Mar-rgo. I go now." She hurried out the door towards the kitchen. I knew she'd clean up my half-finished coffee cup on the way.

I went the other direction and up the stairs to the guest room, where the pillows were perfectly arranged on the bed and the bedspread was pulled snuggly across the mattress—not a wrinkle to indicate a human being had ever slept there. I checked out the blue walls. No cracks, only a few scuff marks here and there. They didn't really need patching or painting, but Margo quite often changed colors on a whim—sometimes her own whim and sometimes her interior decorator's. A paint chip card was Scotch-taped to the wall; the soft yellow color was named "Morning." I took the flat-head screwdriver from my back pocket and began removing the brass faceplates, putting them all together in an empty wastebasket. A few minutes later, Margo poked her head in the room. "Hi, Mike."

"Hey, Margo. How goes it?"

"Okay." But she sounded weary and unconvincing. She stepped into the room wearing a designer workout jacket and pants. She had recently turned forty, but was quite fit and attractive. A personal trainer at the gym and the Wonderbra under her little white T-shirt helped.

"Your sister moved back home, huh?"

She nodded. "Yeah. She and the kids left last week." They had been staying with Margo during her sister's treatment at the USC-Norris Cancer Center.

"How is she?"

She shrugged her shoulders. "It's too early to tell." Sounding like a doctor, she educated me on the billions of cancer cells that had made up the multiple tumors that had forced the removal of both breasts, then maximum chemo and radiation treatments. Her sister's hair had fallen out. She had lost twenty-five pounds.

Trying to give Margo some hope, I told her about Kelly and her new boob.

"That's nice. But it won't save your friend if the cancer comes back."

I got more stuff from the truck, covered the furniture with plastic and the carpet with drop cloths, and prepped the walls. I'd paint them tomorrow and change the lights and assemble the automatic cat box, too. Today, tomorrow, what the hell did it matter? I didn't see Margo or Mariela on my way out, but it was a big house; you could get lost. In the kitchen, I left a note on the island to let them know I'd be back first thing tomorrow. From under the island, the black paw reached out for my pant leg, but its prophylactic nail coverings couldn't hook me.

No one was home when I got there and both kids had rides home from school, so I put on my running shorts and shoes, covered my bare skin with sunscreen, pulled down the bill of my cap, and went for a run. A long run. A very long run. But the melancholy followed me like a dog on a leash: "if the cancer comes back." By the time I got home, it was nearly dark, and my wife's car was parked behind my truck in the driveway. My knee ached again as I climbed our front porch steps. My daughter let me in. She was thirteen and had recently started wearing a bra. They ought to make those damn things cancer-proof. That'd be a Wonderbra.

"Hi, Dad. How was your run?"

"I don't know."

She screwed up her face. "You're so weird."

I pretended to laugh. "It's a gift."

She just shook her head.

"Where's your brother?"

"At the mall with Valerie." My son was seventeen; Valerie was his girl-friend. She drove a hot yellow convertible Mustang, which made my wife uneasy. "Mom's in the kitchen."

I already smelled our dinner on the stove where my wife was cooking a salmon steak in a black frying pan. I leaned against the doorframe, watching her carefully flip the big, red piece of fish with the spatula. Truly, she was a beautiful woman.

"Smells good."

"Oh!" She flinched and looked over at me. "I didn't hear you come in."

"Sorry. Didn't mean to startle you."

She turned to get something from the sink, stopped, stared back at me. "What?"

"What 'what'?"

"What are you looking at me that way for?"

"Just looking."

She eyed me suspiciously, then, as she got nearer, asked, "You *are* taking a shower before dinner?"

I nodded, grabbed a quart bottle of Gatorade—Cool Blue—from the refrigerator, and unscrewed the top.

"Oh, Margo's housekeeper called. Something about an automatic cat box? She said you'd know what she meant."

"Yeah, I know." I took a big gulp of the cold, pale blue liquid, and then remembered, "How soon? How soon?" and I laughed again.

"What's so funny?"

"Ees secret." I took another sip, then, before leaving to shower, leaned against the door frame, and asked my wife, "You busy Saturday night?"

She answered with a question. "Why?"

October Ruse

by H. E. Mantel

You're going to do
What!? *You're sorry!?* You're sorry.
It's been more than 8
years, here, my daughter is twelve,
allowed the in-dignity,

we all do don't we,
blindly, *the crush-cum-pain, but*
in the name of an
authority and trust? You
must seek . . . I did, sought hidden

enemies lumped-in
amongst Nature, *palpable*
you said, yet . . . how few
or many are dead? Betty
came-an'-went, what of Jackie

more, what of she for
herself? *CodePink is not what*
you think, Medea
is the slayer who lets and
quells the flow, you who know but

11

mammo, no!, thermo
is gram positive, chemo
kills, the radio lies
to your bones, the October
rude & ruse, we are the Cure

You want to do what!?
To maim in the name of slash
'n burn, in the guise
of ignorance. You're sorry!?

I am sorry too have to
put this pink ribbon
'round your blue balls in the name
of research & your
mammigrabs, October ride
with the breastless horsewomen

Auntie maims not to
show business, cowed ingénue,
prophylacticized
perhaps, mammodamage for
the good of pharm futures, we

drink at the horsemone
synthqafer, *neigh?!!* Open up
the blinders on the
feed, *You're sorry!? My daughter*
is twelve! *I am the* Cure, *she*

is, we all are in
penis paradise, *Sorry!?*
Tamox'fun no more!

H. E. M.

Cancer Doesn't Hurt

by Kathleen C. Levitzki

I went to see my gynecologist for an emergency visit two days after I found a lump in my right breast. The nurse insisted I come right away because of both the benign lump they had found seven years earlier and the fact that the doctor was leaving for vacation that very afternoon.

They escorted me to an exam room and then simply forgot I was there. It seemed like an eternity sitting in that light hospital robe in mid-August with the air conditioner blasting. My teeth chattering due to the cold and nervousness, I waited for the doctor to hurry into the room to ease my fear. Cancer. I was forty-five. Could I have the same disease that had killed my father at thirty-seven?

Anxiety. I sat there shivering and admitted to myself that I had not felt right for the past fifteen months. I was experiencing a daily fatigue that made getting home from work and making a salad as exhausting as cooking a full Thanksgiving dinner from scratch. I've always watched what I ate and power walked, but when I dropped about thirty pounds I started to eat more calories; it made no difference. I began to lose my sense of smell and taste and could no longer blame it on simply "getting older is really crappy."

I went out into the hall of the office in my thin robe to question the nurse as to the whereabouts of the doctor. About ten minutes later the doctor came in and apologized profusely, adding that my room was only used on an emergency basis and that the nurse forgot to let her know

I had been waiting so long. Her next comment to me was about how thin I had gotten since she last saw me.

Now I was really wondering if they had missed something eight months earlier. She examined me thoroughly and asked many questions. As she pressed my right breast directly on the lump, feeling it, she asked me if it hurt. I said yes it did, very much so. Her response was, "That's good because cancer doesn't hurt." She gave me a prescription for a Fine Needle Aspiration (FNA) with a mammography to follow. Grasping at whatever I could to relieve my anxiety, I took "cancer doesn't hurt" as a comfort.

Two days later I had an appointment at the hospital for the FNA and a mammography. I felt good as I was seeing the chief of the breast cancer center for my needle aspiration. He came in and was very pleasant. After he examined me, feeling the lump that hurt me, he said, "Don't worry; it's going to be nothing."

As he left with the needle and canister containing the cells he had withdrawn, he said he'd be back in less than five minutes with the results. It seemed like he was gone for an hour, but according to my watch it was just four minutes. The moment he walked into the room his happy, smiling face had changed to a very serious and concerned look. He said that there were atypical cells in the biopsy. I asked, "Does that mean I have cancer?" He never answered me and, instead, told me to go to the mammography area. I started shaking and thinking about how to make myself calm enough to go out to the waiting room to tell my husband that I did need the mammography films after all. He was just as scared as me because he knew they were only doing films if there was a problem.

Sitting in the thin hospital gown and waiting for the films brought back the same cold and uncomfortable feelings from the air conditioner that I had felt two days before at the gynecologist's office. When the radiologist walked in and told me that I needed to see a breast surgeon immediately, it hit me that, indeed, cancer does hurt. When I met my husband outside in the waiting room, I was crying. We drove home in fear and silence.

14

Dr. MacIntosh was sweet, soft-spoken, and concerned. She went over all the films with us and took time to answer our every question. The next step was to have the lump removed, so we set up the date of September 11. It was still August; how was I going to wait until September 11 for the surgery? I had no choice. It was her first opening.

When I decided on a mastectomy, Dr. MacIntosh insisted I speak to a plastic surgeon about breast reconstruction. I told her I didn't want any additional surgeries and would simply use a prosthetic breast in my bra. She was adamant, "I will not operate on you unless you see a plastic surgeon first and discuss your options." I didn't want to see another doctor—it was just too much to deal with. Reluctantly, I made an appointment with one of her plastic surgeon referrals, Dr. Sheila Buaond, who convinced me to undergo the breast reconstruction.

After the fear and debilitating effects of chemotherapy and radiation, my greatest crisis was about to happen because of Dr. Buaond's reconstructive surgery. I didn't know it at the time, but this was the beginning of a horror that turned into a miracle.

After the surgery to have saline put into the implant, I had to visit Dr. Buaond's every week. Things weren't going well. I was starting to feel continuous pain on my right side. Dr. Buaond suggested that an infection might be developing and spoke of sending me for an ultrasound to confirm, but she never sent me. She gave me some stronger antibiotics every time I visited, but they weren't working. She continued to speak about sending me for the ultrasound but never gave me the referral.

One day while at work the pain was unbearable. I went into the lady's room and took off my blouse and bra. My right breast, the one that was removed, was totally inflamed and red and felt hot to the touch. The pain radiated through my body to my back. While driving home, I couldn't even lean my back against the driver's seat. Once I got home, I looked at the knives on the kitchen counter in their wooden block and thought about taking the paring knife upstairs with me to cut out the painful implant. Instead, I went upstairs and again took off my blouse and bra. It was a horrid sight. Not only had it gotten a much darker red and much hotter, but the entire shape of my breast had changed. It looked like it had transformed into the Elephant Man's face, and a hematoma was spreading from the bottom of the breast upward. I immediately called Dr. Buaond.

When my husband and I got to her office she seemed horrified, as if realizing she should have sent me for that ultrasound because I had a raging infection. She tried to act calm. She said that she would have to drain the implant. The next bomb she dropped on us was said with what sounded like relief. "I am going away the day after tomorrow on a three-week cruise with my husband. You have to see the doctor who will be covering for me until I return."

His name was Dr. Stafford Broumand. That name should be written in gold capital letters because my miracle was about to begin the following Tuesday. He turned out to be my savior.

My husband and I both left our jobs at lunchtime to meet Dr. Broumand. A nurse took me to an examining room and told me to get undressed from the waist up and gave me a paper robe. Dr. Broumand came in and introduced himself to my husband and me. He was young, soft-spoken, and very kind. He asked me to explain what had been going on and then asked me to open my robe so he could examine me. He tried very hard not to show his dismay at what he saw. He closed my gown, and said, "I have surgery tomorrow, but you are going to leave here now and go across to the hospital and have blood work and a chest X-ray and we are removing this the next day."

He performed the surgery, and then I saw him two or three times for follow up. During my final visit, Dr. Broumand asked me if I would consider redoing the reconstruction after I had healed. I said, "No, never again would I go through this." He said, "You are so young and you won't be happy wearing a prosthesis." I was just so relieved to finally have the excruciating pain disappear and that horrible, deformed breast gone. Dr. Broumand seemed very disappointed but respected my decision. His last words to me were, "You'll be back again."

After having such a severe and life threatening infection, I had to have extremely strong intravenous antibiotics. I wore a prosthesis for the next nine months, which was uncomfortable and painful because of the rampant infection. The minute I would get home from work, I would run upstairs to rip off the bra and prosthesis for some much-needed relief.

Months passed and I became more and more depressed. I knew I needed to speak with someone about all I had been through. After sessions with a therapist, I realized that perhaps Dr. Broumand was correct and that I did need to consider having the reconstruction redone.

I hated the prosthesis; it was a horrible experience for me. I called Dr. Broumand and set up an appointment for a consultation. He was happy to see me again and, of course, I would never consider going back to Dr. Buaond. He went over the entire procedure with me. Again, I felt overwhelmed. Dr. Broumand said, "Go home and discuss everything with your husband; if you need to speak with me further, feel free to call me at any time or come in for another consultation with your husband." Greg and I went back in about a month. We were happy with him and felt secure with his knowledge and ability. We decided to try again.

I was worried that our insurance wouldn't cover another reconstruction. Dr. Broumand is such an incredible physician. He said the law is that they have to pay. He is the medical rarity of a doctor who is more concerned for his patient's well being than lining his pockets with insurance money.

Dr. Broumand's procedures went fabulously and my new breast, nipple, and the tattooing that was done to create an areola came out beautifully. All I could think of was how genuinely happy Dr. Broumand was for me and how this wonderful man made me feel normal again, which really helped my depression.

17

In the operating room, the anesthesiologists were both having a really hard time getting my intravenous fluids started. I was freezing and my teeth were chattering—as anyone who has had surgery knows, the operating room is kept extremely cold on purpose so doctors are comfortable with all their gloves, masks, and lab coats. Dr. Broumand came over to me and held my hand. His hand was so warm and he held mine the entire time they were working on my IV. He held my hand until I fell asleep. His touch was the first thing I remembered when I woke up. What doctor in this day and age does that? When I saw him in the hospital, I told him this and he responded, "Why wouldn't I? You are my patient."

He was so happy, even exuberant, to have made me so happy and satisfied. To me, it seemed as if that was all he needed. He is such a gentle and caring man. Even his staff is above and beyond any staff I have ever worked with. He is so good that he inspires his staff to have his same compassion and uplifting demeanor. Dr. Broumand is young but runs his office with the Hippocratic idealism of an old time practitioner. If he goes on vacation for two weeks, he gets a covering doctor as ethically inclined as himself, in case of any major emergencies. He drives hours to come back one day a week to see his surgery patients. He could just have the covering doctor check the patients, but that is how much he is involved. He wants to examine his surgery patients himself. I asked him about the sacrifice he makes on his vacations; his response was that he doesn't run his practice that way and wants to see his patients himself. I appreciate him so much; there aren't enough words to really express what a wonderful doctor and person he is.

I was thrilled to have this perfect new breast that looked so real. My husband and I just returned from a vacation for the first time since the surgeries performed by Dr. Broumand. What a joy to discover that negative thoughts about my body weren't constantly on my mind during the trip, as well as the utter relief of not having to deal with that horrible prosthesis. I actually bought camisoles and wore them while away.

I even had cleavage in some of the blouses, something I hadn't displayed in years. It finally felt to me as if I were normal again after having gone through so much and feeling so insecure for so long due to gaining weight from certain drugs, wearing a prosthesis, and waiting for my hair to grow back, not in the massive tiny curls that I couldn't do anything with, but to have my normal straight hair back again. All my old clothing was too small for me, and seeing them hanging in the closet was just a constant reminder of what I had lost. What fun it was to go out for dinner that first time on vacation and to actually feel and look sexy. You can't get a better boost than that!

Throughout Dr. Broumand's life he will be praised and awarded by his peers, hospitals, students, and patients. I wanted and needed to write this tribute to Dr. Stafford Broumand so that other cancer patients can feel confident and hopeful that there are, indeed, talented, sensitive, and altruistic doctors out there who will not only heal their suffering and repair their bodies, but also provide the exceptional warmth—be it by holding the hand of a patient on an operating table or by providing gentle words during office consultations—that allows a cancer patient the dignified opportunity to become a proud cancer survivor.

During my first diagnosis, I was told cancer doesn't hurt. That is untrue, but that pain directed me to one of the finest human beings I've ever encountered: my doctor, Stafford Broumand. He made me whole and put the word "happiness" back into my vocabulary.

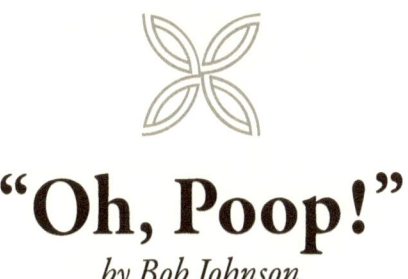

"Oh, Poop!"
by Bob Johnson

In December 2005, I was diagnosed with colon cancer. I was forty-one, which is young for such a diagnosis. After I learned about the diagnosis, I decided to alert my friends and family via email.

One of my priests—I worked at a church—responded to my email with the following:

Bob, you are SUCH a funny writer . . . is there some PLACE for this kind of stuff???? I have NEVER known a cancer diagnosis notification that made me laugh . . . you will BEAT this by sheer HILARITY!!!

This is the email:

From: Bob W. Johnson johnson@stbarts.org

Date: Thu, 05 Jan 2006 13:40:06

To: Friends & Family

Subject: Oh, poop!

Hey y'all!

Hope 2006 has been off to a good start for all of ya. For me, last year ended on a crappy note and the crap continues into the New Year.

On the plus side:
- I've learned what's probably causing the abdominal cramps that have been plaguing me since the end of September (more on that excrement later).

- Move over Anna Nicole Smith! After bouncing back up to my pre-brain-surgery weight, it appears that I'll be entering a Trim Spa type program for which the goal is getting back into my "skinny pants."
- I'll be taking off four to five weeks from work and will be convalescing a hop, skip, and a jump away from the Hamptons!

On the not-so-plus side, it's colon cancer. Here's what I know (I reserve the right to administer poop quizzes):

- The tumor is roughly the size of a petite clementine from Spain.
- The tumor is located in the lower right colon.
- As a bonus, during surgery, my appendix will be coming out, too.
- The surgery is laparoscopic, which means that I will get several small incisions and then my colorectal surgeon will suck the tumor out with a Dirt Devil.
- It doesn't appear to have spread although there may be an unrelated "spot" on my liver. Will know more in the next week or so.
- I'll be going in for surgery (New York Presbyterian/Cornell) on Tuesday, January 17.
- The hospital stay, if there are no complications, will be three to five days.
- No colostomy bag, unless, of course, there are complications.
- Don't know if I will have to endure chemo until after the surgery and lymph nodes have been biopsied. If I do need chemo, Vince and I will be heading to Brooklyn in search of a good chemo wig. Suggestions for good wigmakers welcome.

Here's how we found the tumor:
At the end of September, I had an infected tooth that needed to be extracted. My dentist, Dr. Idyit, had to prescribe an antibiotic to fight the infection:

DR. IDYIT: Bob, do you have any known reactions to antibiotics?

BOB: Yes. Some antibiotics really mess up my digestive tract.

Dr. Idyit prescribed Clindamycin, a drug that is "notorious for causing colitis" (words my colorectal surgeon uttered without any prompting whatsoever!). Bad dentist!

Within two-to-three days the abdominal cramping and persistent diarrhea commenced. Dr. Idyit did not return my calls although I finally reached him three days later:

BOB: I've got cramps. My bowels have gone into overdrive.

DR. IDYIT: Clindamycin wouldn't do that. Something else is wrong with you. Call your doctor.

So I called my doctor's office and filled his nurse in on my leakage problem:

NURSE JILL: You just did a week of Clinda?!

So . . . after a week of Flagyl, then a week of Vancomycin, the cramping and crapping didn't really stop. I decided to take matters into my own hands . . . well . . . you know what I mean . . . and went to see a gastro guy, Dr. Poo. (We like him.)

After a battery of tests (one of which involved a "colon purge"), we ruled out antibiotic-associated colitis and parasites. Last week, during a colonoscopy, Dr. Poo discovered the tumor. Blah de blah de blah.

So there you have it. I'll keep you posted as I learn more. I'll also have my associate, Tara, send out email updates during my hospital stay.

The moral of this story: Although idyit dentists might not know crap about the meds they are prescribing, the incompetence of such idyit dentists could save your life. No shit!

Happy New Year!

Bob

It is now five years later, and I am currently cancer free. I did not need chemo. I did not need radiation. Prayers and laughter can work.

Cancer

by Michael Lewis Jr.

I remember living my life. I was happy
I see my grandchildren laughing and smiling all the time
I wake up each morning pretending that everything is alright
Pleasing my husband and everyone around me
Putting on fronts when actually hurting
Taking care of my grandchildren and not complaining
Enjoying my holidays and the fact that I'm laughing
Everything is ok and I start to wonder:
What will happen if something happens to me?
Who's going to take care of my husband and what about
my grands? My daughter is goin' to make it, but my son . . .
   I don't know . . .

Once I go on vacation everything will work out

All this time I'm Hiding something

Going to the beach, I remember smiling
Walking in the sand, not having a care in the world
Looking into the horizons hoping that there won't be any
   more problems
I'm getting on roller coasters, something I never knew I
   would do
Starting to understand that I haven't done as much as I
   wanted

Remembering my dreams and all my aspirations
I wanted to be an artist but damn that didn't happen
I want to go on a cruise with my family so we can enjoy
    ourselves
Have a big house near my sister so that we can just have girl
    time
Seeing my grandchildren graduate from high school or even
    get married
All these thoughts are coming to me now; why? Is it because
    on the inside I'm a little scared of what might happen
But I'm still on vacation ...

All this time I'm Hiding something

Back now
I've started going to the doctor
Why am I going? Because I have cancer
I start to tear. I don't want to worry my children, but I can't
    keep this a secret any longer
These fronts I put on are starting to dim
I'm getting tired
I just told my kids that I have cancer
They are all worried about me
I don't want them to worry about me; they have to live their
    lives, take care of themselves
I have some regrets though I should've said more
Fought more for what was mine; if I could take back all my
    mistakes, I would

I start chemo today
I feel weak
I get tired easily
I want to sleep
But I have to cook

I have to clean
I have to love
I have to do a lot!
My hair starts to come out
I don't mind. I guess I had a short Jheri curl afro so it's not
    really a big deal
My daughter helps me take the dye out my hair
It's a change, but I'll get used to it

I'm getting sick of this damn chemo
It takes a lot out of me
I never feel like going to the doctor
And for some reason I'm always there
Every time I go to the doctor they tell me things to make me
    feel better
I don't always believe what they tell me, but I just go along
    with it
Since my daughter knows I have cancer, we have really con-
    nected more. I mean, we were close but we're closer now
I can't let cancer bring me down; I can't but for some reason
I think it's going to take its toll and hopefully I'll wind up in
    a better place where I can look down on all of my children
    and protect them for the rest of their lives
And with that I say goodbye!

**A poem written from the perspective of my grandmother,
Clara May Lewis, who died from colorectal cancer on
March 29, 2006.*

27

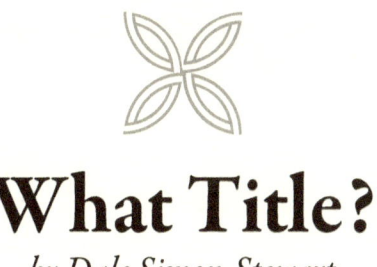

What Title?

by Dale Simon-Stewart

The 2010–2011 academic year began like any other except for one huge, unsettling difference; I was awaiting the biopsy results from my left breast. The day the call came, I was enjoying my first class prep of the day, sitting at my desk correcting essays, and, when I received the news, I would like to say my world tilted. Up to that point my life was wonderfully on track, fantastic family and friends, good health, a son who means the world to me, and a rewarding career that has allowed me to live and work on three continents.

The first flurry of emails I sent out went to my family and my girlfriends here in the USA and those in the UK, South America, and the Caribbean. I was panicking, unusual for me.

After consulting with my doctors and getting the dreaded details and plan of action, my other overriding concern was my son; he was at the mid-point of graduate school. How does one tell a beloved child that everything is not well? Not over the telephone! I enlisted the support of a friend who was a registered nurse, and we both traveled to the University of Connecticut-Storrs campus to tell my son. I felt that my friend would be able to fill in the technical gaps that his father and I were too panicked and unsettled to explain ourselves.

The surgery went well, and my beloved son flew me to Barbados to be with one of my brothers for the recovery period. There with the sun, sea, and surf, I embarked on my very own period of discovery. I discovered why Memorial Sloan Kettering is cited as one of the best facilities treating breast cancer; any concerns I had while recovering were almost instantly addressed via the Internet. My doctors, Cody and Theodoulou respectively, were meticulous, caring, and informative. I discovered that email support is just as effective as real-life interaction when continents separate friends. I discovered that my job as a special education teacher keeps me so busy that I only had a few moments to dwell on my condition. I rediscovered the joys of a small Anglican Church community where my minister is part of my support group. I also discovered that my siblings, who were always asking me to cook meals for them, are great at whipping up meals for me when I am not feeling well. There was only one tiny drawback; my younger brother still refuses to wash up after he cooks.

One surprise discovery was the world of wigs. I am now trying snappy hair styles and colors that I might have never tried without the diagnosis. I was rewarded when one of the eighth-grade boys whom one of my eighth-grade girls thinks is "hot," complimented what he called my "cool look." Finally, I understood why my father nicknamed me "Happy." I am able to stay upbeat and focused on my tilted but still interesting world. For this I am truly humbled and thankful.

I Am a Survivor
by Cetin Otar

I am a survivor, and I'm not going to give up. My Name is Cetin Otar. I had testicular cancer, but now I am a survivor of cancer.

I have been cancer free for about four years now. My experience began when I was seventeen years old. I was a normal student just like everyone else. I was the vice president and co-founder of the student council and I played golf. I was an academically well-rounded student doing his thing to get into college. I also had a girlfriend who was my definition of beautiful. The day it all started is one that I will never forget; it was something that would change my life forever. I told my girlfriend that one of my testicles was larger in size than normal. I didn't think it was serious, but I was mistaken. As time went on, I started having pain in my pelvis; the odd thing was that my testicle went back to its normal size. I told my girlfriend that this had occurred. A couple of weeks later, my testicle swelled again. I really started to worry. I told my girlfriend and she advised me to go see a doctor. I did exactly that.

I went to my physician who referred me to an urologist. I requested the earliest appointment that the doctor had. The doctor told me that it was nothing to worry about and that it was just a bacterial infection. He prescribed antibiotics and told me to come back in a week. A week passed. I went back to the doctor's office. During my check-up, the doctor saw that my testicle had not gone down. The doctor was very puzzled. He started to question himself as to if it might be a tumor. I was traumatized;

I had a hard time believing him. I was given another prescription of antibiotics with a larger dose. The doctor again told me to come back in a week, and I realized that nothing was changing with my testicle. I started to become sick. I had sharp, intense pains like being stabbed with a knife. When the time came to go back to the doctor, I realized that I had been given the wrong appointment date. On top of all that, it was a Jewish holiday, so the office was closed for one week straight; I was screwed.

November 6, 2005, is a day that I will never forget. It was the day that I was rushed to the emergency room because of my testicle. My testicle had grown in mass, so I was rushed to Beth Israel Hospital. That was the hospital where I was told that I would be rushed into the operating room first thing in the morning at 6:30 AM. The first person I called was my girlfriend. I told her about what had happened and she began to cry. My girlfriend told me that she would be there for me from start to finish, and soon after we had gotten off the phone, she came to the hospital. She told me, "Cetin, honey, I want to live a day one less than you so that I will have never, ever, lived a day without you." My first instinct, though I didn't tell anyone, was that I wanted to survive cancer for this girl who loved me, cared for me, and did everything for me.

Everyone I knew around the world found out that I was sick thanks to my mother and the hospital room's phone that she used to call our family in Turkey, my friends, and everyone else. My first reaction to the doctor's remark about me having cancer was very surreal and I was laughing. I started making jokes about the situation while my mother was sobbing on my left and the love of my life sobbing on my right. I concealed the pain that I had inside. On the outside I looked like a brave solider, but deep inside I feared for my life.

The hour came in the morning in which I had to get ready for my surgery. This was round one of my cancer struggle. My operation to remove the tumor inside me was about five hours long. The doctor put in a plastic replacement testicle so that no one would notice it was artificial or even see that I was missing one. When I was out of the operating room, the first things I asked for were my girlfriend and my cell phone. I was really attached to those two things in my life at that point in time.

I was in the hospital for about four days. It was a very painful experience, but I had done it; my first round of the battle was over. I still had the second round to face, but I was somewhat relieved. However, the real hardships had yet to come. We went back to my doctor's office for a checkup the following week; he checked me and explained that he still needed to talk to me about some issues. The doctor told me that the cancer had spread into my lymph nodes, for which I needed to take from six months to one year of chemotherapy. I had absolutely nothing to say to the doctor; I was speechless. While I was listening to the doctor explain the whole process, I faded away into a hole that I had the hardest time getting out of.

After my visit was over, my mom went to a therapist because she was deeply terrified for her baby's life. The therapist told my mother about a doctor at Cornell University Hospital that her mother went to and that this oncologist was one of the best in New York City. My mother's therapist arranged an appointment for me to see this doctor. This was my second opinion. This time the doctor offered an alternative to the chemotherapy: an operation called Retroperitoneal Lymph Node Dissection (RPLND). I didn't know what to do after that appointment and time was running out. That very same day, I went home and my girlfriend and I looked up the operation online. I found out that all of one's organs are taken out and placed in a body bag that is placed on top of the chest as doctors try to get to the location where the cancer has spread. I shared what we had found with everyone in my family. This was the thing that I would have to go through; everyone started to cry.

The second operation wasn't until December 16, 2005. It seemed like that day would never arrive. During this time of waiting, my relationship with my girlfriend was going badly; we were always getting into arguments due to the fact that I was depressed and just wanted to be left alone. She and I would argue about the most ridiculous and mundane topics.

While waiting for my operation, my doctor advised me to go to a sperm bank because he really couldn't tell which lymph nodes were infected; the infected nodes may have been those that allowed me to ejaculate. If they were infected with cancer, he would have to also cut out and clean that area. I wouldn't be able to ejaculate anymore, so I preserved some sperm at the sperm bank just in case.

The day of my operation had finally arrived; we left for the hospital at 4:30 in the morning. I couldn't sleep because I was in a constant state of worry; would it be my last day on this earth and had I had my last supper that night? Would it be the last time I would ever see my loved ones?

We arrived at the hospital around 5:15 AM. I was taken into the back right away because I had to be prepared for my operation. From that point on, it was the hardest time for me because I knew that what I had seen on the computer would all be done to me. I wasn't really upset at anything. I was just feeling lonely, but I had everyone around me that I needed to help me to be strong and brave. As they started getting me ready for my operation with last minute blood work and the like, I started to really let myself relax because I felt something inside of me saying that everything would be alright. I was here in God's world for a test and that this was my test.

Soon after they had my blood work results, they said that I was good to go into surgery, but I had to get one last thing before I went in. They had to install an epidural in my spine. While they were placing the epidural, I felt like I had nothing holding me up any more because the epidural numbed my lower nerve endings so that I wouldn't have pain after the operation. After they had installed the epidural, I was ready to go into the operating room.

They opened the curtains, and I started to walk down to the operating room; the whole family was in tears. I had said goodbye to everyone because, honestly, no one really knew if I would survive the surgery. I couldn't take the fact that I was saying goodbye, so I turned my back to everyone and I started to walk away. On the way to the operating room, I called my girlfriend one last time. I called her to tell her that I really, truly, deeply, madly cared about her and that I loved her with all my heart. She was at home because it was too early in the morning, and I didn't want anything to happen to her. Before we hung up, I heard her start to cry but it was time for me to go. At that moment, I started to pray that my operation would go well. I hopped up on the table and that was it: my moment of truth.

The doctor told me to lie down, so I did exactly what he had requested. The only person who was allowed to come with me into the operating room was my mother. My mom was next to me when the anesthesiologists told her to step outside because the operation was about to begin. My mother said goodbye to me and told me she loved me, kissed me on my forehead, and left the room. I was on my own. As the anesthesiologists placed a mask over my face, I watched my mother leave the room. I started to remember all the great moments that I had lived with my girlfriend, but before I knew it I was knocked out cold. I was in the operating room for ten hours straight. I went into the operating room at 6:00 AM. By the time I was out, it was 3:45 PM. I had exactly seventy-seven staples all lined up one after the other on my stomach. I had made it through my struggle.

When I came back to consciousness, I really didn't know what had happened and before I had the chance to think about it I passed out again. When I awakened, my doctor ordered me to walk around the hospital. That day I wasn't going to be able to walk. I was in pain. I wasn't feeling good. The first couple of days were the most torturous that I have ever had to bear in my life. The second day I tried to get up. That was a big mistake. I fell on the floor trying to get up out of bed. After I fell, I started spewing blood. As a result, I was strapped to the bed so that

I would only walk when the physical therapist, my parents, my cousins, or my girlfriend came to help me.

On the third day, I started to get up by myself but that experience would be just as horrible. I couldn't sleep. I started thinking about committing suicide, jumping out of the window of the hospital or overdosing on drugs, anything so that I could get out of this misery. I used to dread the nights because of my thoughts of suicide, and I couldn't fall asleep because of my heart. A normal human being's hurt beats at approximately 70 beats per minute but mine was beating at 165 per minute. Every night I thought I was going to die. During the day, I didn't feel anything. I just tried to relax in my bed, and when my girlfriend came, I would try to walk around the hospital.

People visited every day. My friends visited, but I cannot recall their visits. I knew that they came by because of the scent left in my room. After I had healed we talked about it and that's how I knew for sure that they had come. Luckily, my mother kept track of who came to the hospital by writing down their names.

I was slowly trying to get back to my normal state. The most that I remember from the hospital time was how my girlfriend, my mother, and my cousin were there for my first post-surgery shower. When I saw everyone working together for my benefit, I felt loved. That shower was the most amazing shower that I had ever taken in my life.

On about the fifth day of my hospital stay, I was allowed to eat. I was allowed to eat only 150 grams of food, but that was a lot of food for me. After I ate, I felt like I had eaten a whole cow.

The days in the hospital had been a whole new experience in addition to the operation. Those days of my life were a nightmare; the whole tragedy was a nightmare for me. I was in the hospital for about seven days. The fact that I was out of the hospital didn't change the fact that I was bedridden in my own home. I had to sleep in my parent's bed because their bed was higher than mine. I could eat only what the doctor told me that I could eat. I had to slowly turn back to life, but, in my head, I was in a whole new world. Those days in my house made me feel as if I were dead. I couldn't move. I had to get permission to be able to do something. They had given me a physical therapist who would come to my house and make me exercise. Every two days the physical therapist would come and push me out of bed to help me to better myself physically. I hated the fact that she would push me out of bed and tell me what to do because I really didn't want to do anything. I didn't want to do anything because I was depressed by everything that was going on with me.

As time went on, the staples in my stomach started to tear my skin apart. I had to go to the doctor's office so that they could take the staples out.

I continued with physical therapy; slowly I started to regain my strength and ability to move freely. The physical therapist told me that I wouldn't be able to do many of the things that I used to. This meant that I would have to be extra careful about how I preformed certain common everyday tasks. I couldn't pick up water basins. I couldn't take showers by myself; I had to be supervised. As a result, I fell more into my depression. I thought I would never be able to move on.

When I was a bit better, I returned to school because I was in my senior year and had only a very short time to apply to colleges. I really wanted to go to American University in Washington DC to become a diplomat, but after I became sick, I changed my mind completely. I wanted to become a doctor. I didn't have that much hope, however; I thought I wouldn't be able to get into any college. I continued in school and when it was time for graduation, I graduated with a 3.7 GPA. I was happy, and before I graduated I had a shot at retaking the SAT. This gave me a little more confidence about actually getting into college. I sent in my scores, but there was no answer until July when my girlfriend called the CUNY office to find out what was going on with my application. They informed her that I had gotten into Brooklyn College and the College of Staten Island. When I heard that I had been accepted into Brooklyn College,

I was extremely happy because it was for the pre-med program. Now I am a junior at Brooklyn College going for my psychology degree.

Dedicated to Reyhan and the whole Otar family and friends.

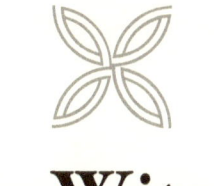

The Witness
by Shell Lewis

It has been a little over four years, and I must admit that it hurts a little less. I didn't think that it could lessen when it first happened. How can losing your mother, watching her die before you very eyes, ever *not* hurt? I was watching *The Witness: From the Balcony of Room 306.* It's a moving documentary centered on Rev. Samuel Kyles, the lone witness to the assassination of Dr. Martin Luther King Jr. Kyles was the only individual on the balcony of the Lorraine Motel with Dr. King on April 4, 1968. Hearing his testimony, I began to cry uncontrollably. Everyone who really knows me will readily admit that I can be a bit emotional. It doesn't take much to make me cry, but it was the particular time at which I watched the documentary that contributed to this spontaneous outpouring of emotion. At the time, I hadn't realized that Rev. Kyles and I also shared something in common. Through the documentary, Kyles hoped to reveal or arrive at the reason why he was chosen to be a witness.

The grieving process takes place through a series of stages and the actual order of the process changes from person to person and situation to situation. I have gone through the initial shock, the denial, the anger, and the acceptance. Now, as I recall the last few months of my mother's life, I wonder why I was chosen to serve as a witness to her death. Why was I chosen over my other three siblings to sit by my mother's side and watch her die?

Every year toward the end of March and the entire month of April, I become a bit melancholy and easily agitated. I have noticed that a similar state takes over my siblings and my aunt around the Easter season too. I watched *The Witness* around this time and figured that it could only be one thing that would cause such an uninhibited reaction. It was my internal alarm clock going off just as it has for the past three years reminding me of the date on which my mother passed, March 29, 2006. It is a date that will truly "live in infamy," at least for me. Even if I do not remember the date, my body innately knows.

I often vividly recall the weeks before Mother passed. She had this pain in her lower spine that wouldn't go away and the pain grew progressively more intense and debilitating; she was bedridden within in a matter of weeks, forced to use a bedpan in her own home. I watched as she would try to get out of bed with either the assistance of my father or myself. Her back spasms became so extreme that her toes would actually curl forward.

"Mommy, your toes are curling underneath your feet."

She never wanted me to think that she doubted her recovery, but I remember her banging her hand against the mattress in frustration, exclaiming in an exacerbated tone, "I just don't understand what's wrong."

It was the first time that I saw doubt on her face. She questioned what was happening to her, and I knew that at that moment she questioned whether she would live. My only response was, "Mom, what's wrong is that you have cancer." I am an emotional person, but I do not believe in sugarcoating. I was and am very blunt, and I, honestly, did not believe that my mother really understood just how sick she was or just didn't want to admit it for the sake of her family. We looked at each other. My mother always took solace in the Lord's word, so I asked if she wanted me to bring her Bible, and, as she tried to position herself in a slightly more comfortable position, she said, "Yes."

As I walked to the living room to retrieve her Bible, it dawned on me that she had been in the bedroom for two weeks and hadn't once asked for it. This was shocking because my mother usually read a Bible chapter a day only to repeat the process when all the chapters had been completed. I grabbed the Bible from the cluttered dining table and walked down the hallway toward her bedroom, stepping across the threshold into the room. As I walked toward her bed, she extended her frail right arm and took the Bible from my hand. As she laid the Bible on the bed and pushed it underneath her so that it would rest directly underneath her lower spine, she said, "Thanks," and turned over to go to sleep.

That's when I called my siblings to let them know the severity of her condition. My parents weren't the best with maintaining personal documents, and I was worried that in the event that something happened none of my mother's paperwork would be in order. I wanted to have everything at hand. My sister planned to visit for a week, just to help out around the house. I still lived at home with my parents and my older brother. My other two siblings didn't know how thin and weak our mother had become, and I wanted them to be prepared for the worse, should it happen.

After a few more days in bed, I began to worry. She shouldn't have stayed at home in that condition. We weren't medically equipped to alleviate her pain, and my father, with all good intentions at heart, began to overmedicate my mother. He hated to see her in pain and, although I was changing her pain patch according to directions and seeing to it that she took all other necessary pills, he would give her an additional patch when I was away. I came home on one occasion, opening the door with my key as I yelled down the hall, "Mom, I'm home." I didn't get a response. I walked into the living room where my father rested in his recliner. He told me that she may be asleep, so I went into her room and proceeded to speak to her. Her speech was slurred and she spoke incoherently; every so often her eyes would roll back into her head. I thought the worse but something told me to examine her body for additional pain patches and I removed two patches that I found and attempted to make her drink a lot of water so that I could flush the drugs out of her system.

I went to my father and explained that he cannot give her additional pain patches, that he must follow the package directions and that he can cause her to overdose. She was on way too many pills for him to do something as foolish as upping her dose or mixing pain medications without doctor approval. He looked at me and began to cry. I knew he didn't mean to cause her any harm.

"Dad, you have to be strong. You cannot let her see you cry. If she thinks you have given up, what do you think she will do?"

A few more days had passed and both my mother and I had agreed that if her condition hadn't improved, I would call her oncologist and request that an ambulance pick her up and take her to the emergency room. My father disliked the idea; he was under the impression that she would be sent back home. Since she wasn't improving, I called her doctor and explained that she had been in the bed for two weeks and that she could not get up without assistance. I added that she had such severe back spasms that her toes would curl forward, underneath her feet. The oncologist thought that she may have had a stroke and agreed that she needed to be admitted for further examination.

"A stroke?" I said to myself. I really didn't think that she had had a stroke. Either the cancer had spread or something else was going on.

I told my mother that the ambulance was on its way. She immediately told me to wash her up. I filled a washbasin with warm water and, while she lay in bed, proceeded to give her a sponge bath. The water was too cold for her so she grimaced. I attempted to move with as much haste as possible so that she wouldn't have to lay undressed for long. Since she couldn't move without experiencing a spasm, we struggled to get her dressed. She placed all her upper body weight on her elbows, forcing them into the mattress, so that she could raise her lower half as high as possible while I pulled a pair of loose fitting lounge pants up securely around her waist. We were able to get a clean shirt on with fewer theatrics.

The ambulance came, equipped with two young EMTs who were incredibly kind. They asked what had happened, and I explained that my mother has cancer, adding that she couldn't get out of bed. They both headed to the bedroom and spoke to my mother to confirm her condition and then they both headed back up the hallway to where I stood. I held the door while they rolled the stretcher down the hall to my mother's bedroom. It's bizarre, but I cannot recall exactly where my father was during this time. He was in the apartment but for some reason, I cannot remember exactly where. Once my mother was lifted from her bed to the stretcher, we were on our way.

The ride to Cabrini Medical Center in Manhattan was incredibly bumpy. My mother winced in pain as the ambulance plowed over every pothole. It was as if the jolts sent electrical shocks through her spine. I had never seen her have such a reaction. We finally arrived at the emergency room. My mother had been in and out of the hospital for several weeks, staying for one-to-two week intervals at a time. I had grown way too familiar with Cabrini Medical Center and honestly didn't care to be within its walls. I'm not saying that the staff was incompetent or lacking in any particular ability. I was just tired of the hospital and all things associated with the medical practice. My mother was immediately given steroids, which eased her pain almost instantly. She actually bent her legs toward her chest and didn't notice the involuntary movement. My father and I simultaneously pointed it out to her.

She was admitted into the hospital so that her doctor could find the right combination of drugs to ease her pain. She couldn't stay on steroids, though, I must admit, they definitely did the job. While taking them, she was able to move around as if she wasn't even sick.

Her oncologist was a round, middle-aged Russian woman with the very best of intentions but the idea that she couldn't provide any answers, and the way she actually looked puzzled when I described my mother's state made me feel incredibly uneasy. At the time, my mother had a surgical oncologist who was simply fantastic. I called him up when her routine oncologist couldn't provide any answers.

After I described my mother's condition, the surgical oncologist thought that the problem seemed neurological and informed me that he was going to place his colleague, a critical care doctor, in charge of her overall medical care. My mother was actually released from the hospital shortly after we spoke, per her oncologist's approval. I wasn't aware that she was released when I spoke with the surgical oncologist.

My mother was at home for about two weeks before I had to call to have her readmitted. It was about three weeks after I had spoken with my siblings and my sister planned to drive up from Georgia that weekend.

I was at Brooklyn College and had just wrapped up my shift at the Brooklyn College Learning Center, which is where I worked while earning my graduate degree. I was standing outside of Boylan Hall, conversing on my cell with my sister-in-law about my mother. My mother's appetite had long since dissipated, but she would force herself to eat a few bites to maintain her strength. While in the hospital, she simply refused to eat and, as a result, she wasn't given her medication. Thinking about it now, she should have been fed intravenously. She hadn't even received her chemo treatments in over a month because her Port-a-Cath became clogged, which was something that I had grown accustomed to. If the Port-a-Cath worked as it was expected, then her blood work wasn't at the permissible levels to receive treatment. It was always something!

Needless to say, my mother's disposition changed for the worse. The doctor who the surgical oncologist called to take over her medical care dropped by and spoke with my mother and I as my father listened in on the conversation. He asked my mother about her symptoms and what she was feeling and reassured us all that he would get down to the bottom of the matter. He spoke with me outside of her hospital room. He didn't beat around the bush and neither did I. He told me that he believed that the cancer had spread to her bones, specifically to her lower spine, which was causing her back spasms and related complications. He added that he planned to have X-rays made to confirm his speculations so that he would know exactly what additional areas needed to be treated and that she would have to have targeted radiation treatments in addition to chemotherapy.

"Will you be able to treat the area so that it will no longer be an issue?" I asked.

He assured me that he would and that he would then have to place her on a pharmaceutical regime that would treat all her conditions and symptoms: colorectal cancer, a propensity for blood clotting, high blood pressure, and liposarcoma, another form of cancer that had developed shortly after her first surgery. I appreciated his honesty and the fact that he provided me with some answers. The X-rays were taken.

It was Monday, and I went to visit my mother as soon as I was dismissed from class. My mother was contemplative. The television was on but she wasn't paying much attention to the characters that paraded back and forth on the screen. She kept looking at the door. I couldn't figure out what had captured her attention.

"Is that a chapel?" she asked, turning her head to face me. "It looks just like a church."

"No. It's just a wood door," I replied. I looked at the door and noticed that the natural finish caused the illusion of a lopsided steeple. From the corner of my eye, I noticed that my mother was now intently gazing at me. She was satisfied with my response. I could tell from the way she replied with a resolute "Okay!" I let her look at me for a moment. It was as if she was taking it all in, taking me all in. I turned to look at her and she looked me in the eyes and smiled. I asked what was wrong and she simply replied, "Nothing." She continued to look at me for a bit more, still smiling, and then turned her head to watch the television.

I recall my father stepping into the room at this time. He had been searching for a parking spot in the area and had just arrived. When my mother saw my father, she yelled out, "Hi!" Perhaps it was my father's expression that sticks out so vividly. He greeted her with the same degree of enthusiasm but tinged with astonishment. My mother hadn't greeted anyone in such a manner in months. Once my father had gotten settled, I decided it was time for me to head home. I was pursuing my MA in English and had to draft a paper for the following day. I also had to open the Learning Center in the morning. I told my mother goodbye and that I loved her. She replied, saying "I love you too."

On Tuesday, March 28 it was like déjà vu. I was again standing in front of Boylan Hall speaking to my father. I had called my mother's room and he picked up the phone.

"Hi, Daddy. Can I speak to Mom?"

"She's in the bathroom," my father replied.

"What? Did she walk by herself to the bathroom?" I asked.

"Yeah. She did but she doesn't feel well. I gotta go. She's coming out and I gotta help her," my father said before hanging up the phone.

I thought that this was a sign of improvement. She hadn't walked for about a month. I immediately got on the phone and called my sister-in-law and my sister, telling them both that Mom had walked, by herself, to the bathroom and, given the news that her critical care doctor had provided, we were all under the impression that things were about to turn around. I made it to Manhattan that night too late to visit the hospital. I decided not to call my mother's room because it was a little after nine and she would either be asleep or about to go bed. Anyway, I would be at home soon and my father would inform me of any change, if necessary.

When I opened the apartment door, my father was in the kitchen. He seemed both simultaneously elated and discouraged. She really felt bad, but, nevertheless, she had walked, he said, sprinted, even, to the bathroom.

46

After a brief conversation, we both went to bed. For the first time in several weeks, I slept soundly.

On Wednesday, March 29, 2006, I awakened a bit earlier than usual that morning. I had to open the Learning Center; I had the keys to the Center in my possession. My father was already up. He was about to make his daily visit to the hospital and was getting dressed in his bedroom. My eldest brother was in the back room with his two kids. I was about to put on my shoes when the phone rang. I sprinted to the living room and picked up the phone.

"Lewis residence."

"Hello, this is Dr. Jefferson, the resident doctor at Cabrini Medical Center . . ."

My heart sank.

"May I speak with Mr. Lewis?" he asked.

"This is her daughter; you can tell me," I replied.

"I'm sorry ma'am, but Mrs. Lewis passed away this morning."

I wasn't shocked. I cannot really explain what I felt. I guess from serving as the liaison between my mother, her doctors, and both the immediate and extended family and friends, I felt a simultaneous sense of relief and inexplicable pain. Dr. Jefferson informed me that she had apparently passed during the night and they weren't quite sure what had taken place.

"You have to tell my father," I explained. I asked the doctor to hold on while I went to get my father.

"Daddy, you gotta come to the phone."

"Why? Oh, God. What happened?" he cried as he ran toward the living room and picked up the receiver. Shortly after holding the phone to his ear, he dropped the receiver, banging his hands against the recliner, rocking it violently back and forth. I picked up the phone and asked the doctor what would happen now. My mother was the one who normally would have handled such a situation. He informed me that her body was going to be taken to the morgue and that I would have to contact a funeral home to retrieve the body. I asked him if he would be able to keep the body in the room so that my siblings, my father, and I could see her. He said that he would hold the body in the room for as long as he could. At that moment, I was hoping it was a mistake and that when we arrived at the hospital, we would find that it wasn't Mom who had passed. We would find out that there was some mix-up.

The first person I called was my mother's sister. I told her what had happened, and I was shocked by how calm she was. She was definitely upset. Both of her parents had passed and it was just her and my mother, but her tone was one of acceptance. It was the reaction that I would have expected from my mother, that calming affirmation that everything would be okay and that you knew what it is that you must do. I explained to my aunt that I needed to call everyone and she said, "Okay." I called my sister and told her that Mom had died. She began to scream and I couldn't make out what she was saying. The phone went dead.

I proceeded to call my brother who lived on Staten Island; he was driving when I called. He had just gotten off from work.

"Michael, Mommy died."

"What?"

"Michael, Mommy died."

"What did you say, Shell?"

"Michael, Mommy died, and I need you to get over here right now because I don't know what to do . . ."

I couldn't contain my emotions any longer. I started to sob uncontrollably and my brother told me to hang up the phone. He called his wife, and they removed their children from school and headed to the hospital. I managed to call my sister-in-law and asked her to inform by brother that the doctor wasn't sure how long he would be able to keep my mother's body in the room.

My father and I then drove to the hospital. My father had calmed down a bit. I suppose because he was driving, he realized that he needed to stay calm.

It wasn't yet visiting hours and the security guard stopped me before I reached the elevators, "Where are you going? You cannot go upstairs yet."

"My mother just died. I have got to go upstairs. Please just let me go upstairs."

He apologized for my loss and ushered me into the elevator. My father and eldest brother were with me. My other brother and his family were driving from Staten Island.

When we arrived in her room, I realized that it was true, for she was already in a body bag. They attempted to mask the bag from which her body partially protruded with bed sheets. They had removed the socks that she had on her feet and all her clothes, exposing the Port-a-Cath that hadn't worked in over a month. All of her belongings were consolidated into a used paper bag: her eyeglasses, Bible, undergarments, and clothes. Her eyes were fixed on the ceiling, her mouth agape.

The clothes that were in the bag were moist; feeling how damp her socks were, I couldn't even begin to imagine what had taken place during the night. I just knew that her last night on this earth wasn't a pleasant one.

It is cliché but true; watching my mother die could have honestly killed me, maybe not physically but it could have very well killed me emotionally. I went through a lot while my mother was sick and took on the responsibilities that she tended to while in good health. I cooked, cleaned the house, kept my family informed of my mother's condition, served as a liaison between my mother and her doctors, worked part-time, and attended graduate school. After my mother passed, I took over her household bills until I moved out and into my own apartment. The entire experience prepared me to take care of myself, and I am a stronger person largely due to witnessing my mother's death. It's morbid but, nevertheless, true.

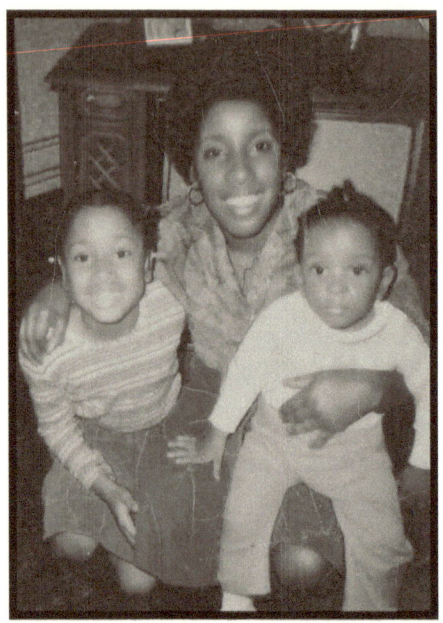

Clara and her two daughters,
Sharon (left) and Shell (right).

My Name Is Prasenjit Chandra

by Prasenjit Chandra

I live in Calcutta, the cultural capital of India. I am forty years old. I graduated with an engineering degree in 1992. I am married and living with my family. I have my mother, brother, my wife, and nine-year-old son. My father also was the victim of Renal Cell Carcinoma. He was diagnosed in September 2008 and died in December 2008. From childhood, I often had sores on my tongue. They would disappear when I took medicine or coated them with ointment. In August of 2004, there was a white sore that appeared on the left side of my tongue. Prior to the appearance of the sore, one of my teeth broke and a portion of my tongue continuously touched the broken tooth. I applied medicine, but the wound would not heal; rather, it was getting bigger. I read an article about oral cancer. I rushed to an oral pathologist. She recommended some medicine and asked me to come again after one month. After one month, when she saw no improvement, she suggested a biopsy. Hearing that word, "biopsy," I felt very nervous. I went to the most respectable homeopathy doctors. They assured me that they were able to cure me. I wasted more than eight months with them. When there was no improvement, I again consulted with the oral pathologist. She reviewed the biopsy. On the 31 of May, 2005, I got the results, which were positive; it was Squamous Cell Carcinoma. She suggested surgical removal of the lesion. Then I consulted an oral and maxillofacial micro vascular surgeon, who performed my ten-hour-long operation on the 11 of June, 2005, at a nursing home in Calcutta. Half of my tongue was removed and then reconstructed from the tissue of my left hand.

After three months, I returned to a normal life. I regularly go to the doctor for checkups, blood tests, an Ultrasonography (USG) of my neck and my whole abdomen, and X-rays every six months. Now I am leading a normal life with my family, but all my family members, including myself, are always tense because we don't know when and in what form the disease might return. I am always worried, believe me. I lead a completely normal life and when I am at work, I always try to forget that I had cancer, but it is very hard, very tough, and it is always in my subconscious mind, which is much more disturbing than the disease itself.

If treated at an early stage, cancer is not incurable. Basically for head and neck cancers the success rate is 80 percent if treated at the first stage. Now there are treatments, such as radiation and chemotherapy, for the later stages, too. The treatment helps the victim to live much longer and feel less pain. In my case, I am grateful to the Almighty for an early detection and the right treatment. I am grateful to my family, especially to my father; without their support, I would never be normal. I am also grateful to the doctors who treated me with the best intentions and the appropriate form of treatment.

I am living a whole new life, and I want to live this God-gifted new life in a completely different way. My new life is dedicated to making only good in the society. I saw death very closely as I was near it. When someone is near death, only he or she can explain his or her feelings; those who know their fate must think differently. Generally, a healthy person thinks only of his own problems and his family, but a cancer survivor thinks about more than that . . .

As a cancer survivor, I will always advocate for a smoke-and-tobacco-free world. In India *guthka* and *pan masala* (chewing tobacco products) are very popular. Most people aren't aware that *guthka* and *pan masala,* are the main cause of oral cancer in India. I want to do something good for poor cancer patients. The condition of poor cancer patients is horrible. Family members, knowing full well about the condition of their loved ones, spend a lot of money for treatment by selling their houses, ornaments, and fertile land and even by borrowing money at high interest rates. As a result, the family is the worse off after the death of their loved one.

As a survivor, I am doing something for them, but I have limitations as I don't have many funds, and I am not aware of any organizations that might be able to provide assistance. I am seeking advice from the readers.

If you can help, please contact me at:

Prasenjit Chandra
Flat No.: 401
36/3, South End Park
Calcutta 700029
West Bengal
India
Email: prasenjitchandra@yahoo.com

Tub Thumping
by Carol Ann Pretzel

Remember Chumbawumba? They had a real catchy tune back in the fall of '97: "Tub Thumping." Technically, I think it was about going on a British drinking binge, but it was a real upbeat song. At the time I was working at a brain-injury rehabilitation center in Boston, The Greenery, in the recreation department, and it was around Halloween. As my coworkers and I decorated the recreation room for the annual Halloween party, we'd crank the radio way up while we blew up orange and black balloons and draped matching colored crepe paper from one end of the room to the other, including the physical therapy equipment. "Tub Thumping" was being played a lot those days, and I'd quit what I was doing and go into a (very) lame attempt at dancing, but it gave the residents who happened to be rolling by (most of them were in wheelchairs) a good giggle.

It was the chorus that really spoke to me: "I get knocked down, but I get up again; you're never gonna keep me down." I've always identified with the underdog, trying but never quite making it, having good ideas but never at the right time, and getting knocked down then picking up my poor old butt and movin' on.

I had been working at The Greenery for a little over a year. I couldn't think of a better job than what I was doing—having fun helping others to have fun. It could be tiring sometimes but it was worth it, and I had a great team of coworkers. The next big event we had after Halloween was the Holiday Flea Market and Craft Sale. If I thought decorating for Halloween was a little tiring, setting up everything for this event was much worse. Finding, folding, and carrying those long tables into the hallway on the main floor and setting up the goodies—everything from residents' crafts to my crafts, yard sale stuff, and delicious baked goods—was quite a task. Thank goodness we had some volunteers to help out because I was really dragging during the sale itself. One thing I can remember was a hangnail on my right-hand thumb. I chewed and pulled it off—nerves, I guess—and it started bleeding a little. It would scab over some but, then, at the least bump, start bleeding again. It's weird, some of the minutiae that sticks in your brain: that lousy hangnail.

As I mentioned earlier, my attempts at dancing were quite dorky at best. I'm not the most graceful girl on the block and would bump into my shadow if given half a chance, so I wasn't too concerned to see black and blue marks sprout up on my arms and legs. Hey, I'm sure I banged myself around quite a bit moving those tables. Not only was I clumsy, but I had a propensity to bruise easily, so like I said, it was no big whoop. My husband, however, saw it differently. I couldn't be that clumsy. I had bruises on my arms and legs, on the inside of my legs, too. They were two quite large designs in a lovely shade of purple. It looked like my husband had whacked me around some, but that was the furthest thing from the truth. He wanted me to tell my doctor about it. "No rush," I said. I'd see her in a couple of weeks anyway for my yearly exam, and I'd bring it up to her then. In between then and the visit I made a very crude drawing of where these black and blues were located.

I still have that drawing.

I was living in Massachusetts at the time, right on the New Hampshire border, and my doctor was in Nashua, New Hampshire, about a twenty-minute drive away. The exam, a routine Pap test, went OK. After I got dressed and was getting ready to go I remembered about the bruises and my promise to my husband to ask about them. She looked at them—although how she could've missed the ones on my inner thighs when she did the initial exam is beyond me—and didn't think it was anything to be concerned about but decided to take some blood for a workup anyway.

Twenty minutes later I was home and watching reruns of *The Simpsons* when the phone rang. It was the doctor. My blood work looked kind of strange, and she wanted to know if I could drive up to St. Joseph's Hospital in Nashua so that another sample could be taken. She'd made all the arrangements and asked me to hang around at the hospital for a while for the results to come in. Sure! I left a little note for my husband who wasn't home from work yet, hopped into the car, drove to Nashua, had some more blood sucked out of my arm, and sat and waited until my doctor called. She was very worried, concerned that my "platelet" count was very low. (My *what?* I thought they were little dessert plates.) She was so concerned, in fact, that she admitted me into the hospital then and there. I felt fine—what was I doing in a hospital? I was led to my room, and, not having had supper yet, I requested a turkey sandwich, which came without enough mayo. (There's that recollection of minutiae again!) I called Barry, my husband, who was home by now, and asked him to pack my toothbrush, deodorant, and a change of undies for me and bring them up.

My doctor finally came in and explained why she was concerned. Platelets are the stuff that helps your blood to clot. In some cases, like mine, with a platelet count this low a person could easily bleed to death from the inside, and she wanted to make sure that didn't happen to me.

But I felt fine!

The next morning I met another doctor, a hematologist, who looked at my feet, which were generously sprinkled with tiny freckle-like pinpoints. I had noticed them before but hadn't thought much about them. Hey, they were my feet! But those little marks were petechia, not a very good sign. I made arrangements to see my doctor for some more blood tests and was discharged. (I recall that it was snowing that day.) I don't remember how many times I went to have my blood taken but they couldn't determine what was wrong by just doing that. I needed a bone marrow biopsy, which is something that I won't go into right now except to say it wasn't a whole lot of fun. Then the waiting began.

In the meantime, I went to New York City, specifically the Bronx, to spend Thanksgiving with my in-laws. I took a photo of my father-in-law carving the turkey with the same scowl on his face he has every year when he does it. I have the photos to prove it. After coming home, I talked to the hematologist who said there was something going on, but he didn't have the final results. We scheduled an appointment with my primary doctor in about a week.

On Monday, December 8, 1997, it was a chilly, overcast day when I went back to see my doctor. When she put her arm around my shoulder and led me into her office instead of an exam room, I knew something wasn't quite kosher. After we sat down she dropped the bomb: I had leukemia. Acute Myelocytic Leukemia (AML) is a very rapid, often fatal form of the disease. The word "leukemia" rattled around in my brain like a ball in a pinball machine—the old fashioned kind. "It's got to be a joke," I thought. My doctor told me that I actually had Acute Promyelocytic Leukemia (APML or APL to those of us who came to know it intimately), a subtype of AML that she was unfamiliar with because it wasn't very common. How long did I have? With AML, maybe six months if untreated. I felt so alone there all by myself in my doctor's office in Nashua, New Hampshire while Barry was at work in Worcester, Massachusetts, over an hour's drive away. I had to tell him.

I called the law office where he worked, but he wasn't there; he was at the law library. It was *really* important that I talk with him as soon as possible, I told one of the partners. Would he be able to get Barry back to the office for me? I gave him my doctor's private number. Barry called. I got on the line with the doctor and she told him the news. I really do not remember what his reaction was or if I cried when I told him. It's funny. I can tell you how much mayo had been on a sandwich but not what our reactions were.

Before leaving the doctor's office, she called the Dana-Farber Cancer Institute in Boston and made an appointment for me to see one of its best leukemia specialists, Dr. Richard Stone. I took the card that she had written the information on and left her office. Yes, I was OK to drive home. It was dark out; the sun was setting quite early at that time of year. It was snowing, not a lot, but enough to make itself known and cause one to take extra precautions when driving. It really isn't such a smart idea to be driving at night, in the snow and crying, but what the hell . . . if I only had six months.

"I get knocked down, but I get up again" The radio was talking to me. Well, singing to me, actually. I felt a little resolve as I heard the song, but the word "leukemia" kept interrupting Chumbawumba. What had I done to get leukemia? I didn't smoke, drink a lot, hang around toxic chemicals. Why? And why me? After arriving at home, all I could think about was that I wouldn't get to see the turn of the century or turn fifty years old.

When Barry came home, we had a good cry. Well, I did anyway; he was very reassuring that it would be OK. Hah! Easy for him to say when he wasn't the one with cancer flowing freely through his veins! We called his folks. Mine had passed away about eight years earlier, and I was grateful they wouldn't have to be around to see me die. We called my aunt and uncle, who were the only immediate relatives I had that I was close to. When she found out, a cousin called to see if it was hereditary. (It's not.) Then we hit the Internet to learn all we could about APML.

The visit to the Dana-Farber Cancer Institute went well. My doctor was a tall, goofy kind of guy, but he knew his stuff. He gave me encouraging news; although it was an acute leukemia, the fact that it was APL worked in my favor. He had recently attended a symposium on the West Coast about the drug the Chinese are using on APL patients: All-Trans Retinoic Acid (ATRA). That, combined with chemotherapy, gave me an 80 percent cure rate. Sounded a lot better than six months to me! He gave me the choice of being admitted to Brigham and Women's Hospital that night or the next day. I chose the next day so we could enjoy a last dinner out, and I could finish addressing the Christmas cards.

That night, as usual, we watched David Letterman on TV. I really liked Letterman—still do. I had hoped to see him live some day, but I guess that wasn't in my future. Dave usually has a musical guest on towards the end of the show. That night, it was . . . Chumbawumba. "I get knocked down, but I get up again." Something pinged inside my brain, but this time the tears were ones of determination. This was one weird coincidence to be hearing this song, with its upbeat chorus, the night before I was to enter the hospital for what might be the most trying time of my life up until then. I was going to be the one getting back up again, damn it!

To make a long story short,—OK, so it's too late for that now—while I was lying in bed having all sorts of strange stuff pumped into me through a catheter in my chest, I'd get phone calls from my co-workers. No words, just, "I get knocked down, but I get up again." They held the department Christmas party in my room, but because my white blood count was next to nothing and my immune system nearly kaput, the rec director needed to wear a mask because she had a cold. But I have to say, pizza and Diet Coke never tasted so good. The chemo didn't make me sick, but my hair did fall out, every single strand, all over my body. (Hey, washing my "hair" was a breeze now, and I wouldn't have to worry about "hat hair" or shaving my legs!) The Greenery administrator stopped by and gave me copies of *Don't Sweat the Small Stuff* and *The Perfect Storm*. Some of my coworkers from other departments spent their time off donating platelets and blood, which I went through like Kool-Aid.

I spent the Christmas of 1997 in my room on the seventh floor. Barry decorated it with Christmas cards, a small fake tree, and a string of tiny lights. Flowers and fresh fruit were prohibited. I also experienced 1997 turning into 1998 there, watching a monster movie marathon on TV,—Lord, how I love 'em!—dozing in and out of consciousness, snacking on the burnt Chex Mix that Barry had made, and toasting the New Year with grape ginger ale while watching Dick Clark's Rockin' New Year's Eve Show. A little after midnight, do you know who came on and what they sang?

"I get knocked down, but I get up again, you're never gonna keep me down"

My doctor said I was in remission on January 28, 1998. For the next few years we drove to Boston every few months for a blood test and bone marrow biopsy. Then we'd go and do something fun, like eat out and go to the movies. It's really amazing that I can remember this much since the medication I took before the biopsies and all during my chemo had the side effect of wiping out a lot of my short-term memory. When we'd get home, I'd have to ask Barry, "What did the doctor say? And what did I say? Did you say anything?" One really cool thing was that in the summer when all the reruns were on TV, they were "new" to me, because I couldn't remember seeing them the first time because I was in the hospital!

Our trips to Boston continued, even after we moved to Maine. In fact, my last visit to see my doctor was on September 11, 2001. Amid all the chaos and horror that was on the TV in the lobby of the Dana-Farber Cancer Institute, I was beaming in the exam room when my doctor declared me "cured."

While I was in the hospital, I went through a lot of denial. This must be some really elaborate practical joke someone's playing on me. OK, you can stop now. But he didn't, and a year later it was all like a dream, like it never even happened. But I have pictures of a very bald me to prove that it did. (Mother Nature was kind to me. I didn't have any unsightly bumps or ridges on my head!) I was very lucky. Even now, when I put it on the stereo or catch a radio station playing it when I'm in the car, I get a lump in my throat, tear up a little bit, and feel real good when I hear, "I get knocked down, but I get up again."

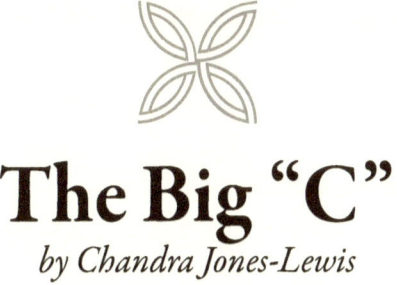

The Big "C"
by Chandra Jones-Lewis

Umm, that could mean anything: the big candy, the big cookie, the big piece of cake. Ladies and gentlemen, I'm not talking about some damned sweet treat; I'm talking about CANCER.

Wow, I can't believe I've been touched by this twice. First my aunt Blanche died, then my mother-in-law, Clara. Both times have taken me by surprise. Am I being naïve? Did I really know and not want to face reality? No, no, no! I was taken by surprise and that's final. I can't quite remember the correct order of events that led to such sorrow, but here it goes:

- The beach house vacation
- While on vacation, whisperings about something being wrong
- Family back from vacation
- Doctor appointments
- Tests
- Diagnosis, diagnosis, diagnosis

I'm not sure who told me first. Was it my husband? Was it my sister-in-law, Shell? I do remember calling my uncle to tell him because my aunt died of the same thing and his response was, "son of a bitch."

- Calls being made and lots of discussion among family members
- Constantly on the phone with Shell

I could go on and on to describe all the calls, but I won't. As you can imagine, the telephone lines were burning up because all we could do was talk about it with one another. I guess it was an early form of therapy for all of us.

Note: the following is definitely out of order.

- Call from Shell. Positive news; the doctor said they will start Mom on solid food soon.

- Husband tells me he has to take Mom to a doctor's appointment, and his dad keeps calling him to make sure he doesn't forget. (Who knew this would be his mom's last ride in his truck?)

- My mom and I going to the hospital to visit her. I didn't realize how much weight she lost.

- Call from Shell saying Mom really wasn't feeling well and she's in a lot of pain.

I don't remember how much time passed before I had this brief conversation with Henry, my brother-in-law.

Henry: Poo (my nickname), is Mike home?

Me: No Hen; what's up?

Henry: Mom died.

Me: Oh my god, oh my god!

Phone line goes dead.

- Pick up Michael from school.

- Drive to hospital, long, dazed, silent.

- Mom on bed, small and cold.

- Body bag!

- Left hospital to make arrangements.

- Day or two later, viewing of body.

- Car ride to South Carolina.

- Funeral!

My husband was extremely angry. He's still angry. His mother's death has been very hard on him, as have all the events that happened afterward, but I won't begin to get into that. He has so many unresolved issues with his mom. The issues will always be unsettled because she's gone, but I'll be there to love him, and I'll be there when he wants to talk about her.

Present day

My children don't talk about their grandma much, but they do have memories of her. My son, Michael, remembers the most.

Even though this happened years ago, we all speak of it as if it could have been yesterday. All of the conversations we had together are so fresh in our minds. I'm still learning things I didn't know before. It's gotten easier to talk about, but I know the family will never get over such a huge loss.

Rest in Peace, Clara

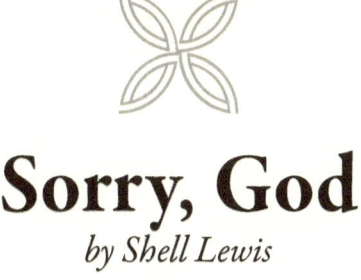

Sorry, God

by Shell Lewis

I have never been at a loss for words. I've always been able to articulate my feelings, to express my sentiments, but my pain is so deep, so incredibly deep that all words meet and crowd in my throat, rendering me incapable of speaking as I choke on my own grief.

I miss my mother!

I miss the beam of light that I was blessed to have known, if only for twenty-seven years. I can truly say that I was blessed to have been the physical Clara May's daughter, and I am even more blessed to be the angelic Clara May's daughter.

This piece is dedicated to all those who expressed their condolences by exclaiming, "God knows best" and "It was God's will." I have several qualms with these consolations. Let us consider what these sentiments really express. Basically, what I was told on numerous occasions was that God wanted my mother to have colon cancer and that God wanted my mother to have surgery during which sizable portions of her colon and left ovary were removed along with surrounding lymph nodes. God wanted her to lose all of her hair, her appetite, and strength due to chemotherapy and radiation treatment. God wanted her to have yet another operation and develop second degree burns below her left knee from a second bout of radiation to treat the liposarcoma that had materialized months before in the treated area. God wanted her to fall face-first on the pavement due to what I speculate was the spread of the disease into her bones.

(Unfortunately, my mother did not live long enough for examination results to confirm my speculation.) God wanted her to develop a blood clot in her left leg as a side effect of surgery. God wanted her to take blood thinners for the remainder of her life to prevent the reoccurrence of a clot. God wanted her to develop a cancerous lesion on her lower spine. God wanted her to die in a hospital bed with her mouth agape and eyes fixed in one direction as if she saw death approaching.

"I am so sorry," they said, adding, "but it was God's will," which equates to "I am so sorry but God wanted your mother to suffer and then die." I refuse to believe that God would want anyone to suffer in such a manor. I refuse to believe that the same God my mother cherished would inflict such pain on his loyal servant. (Yes, my mother was God's loyal servant!) What I cannot seem to understand is why people do not think before they speak. Why is it that they really don't consider what they're saying and what their words really mean? God does work in mysterious ways. This I believe is true, but there are two forces at work in the world and this seems more like the latter's doing.

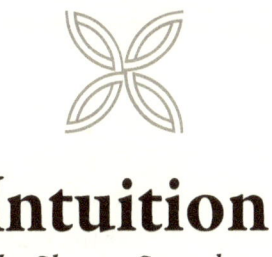

Intuition

by Sharon Saunders

I had the oddest dream. Beautiful flowers filled the room. She was so dissat-isfied with them. "Why do these flowers disappoint you?" I asked. She shook her head in disapproval. I explained to her that the flowers were only kind gestures from people who cared about her. I smiled at her. She appeared so uneasy about what was happening. I didn't comprehend the meaning of it.

Did You Hear?

I remember the phone call. My mother said, "I don't want you to get upset; I went to the doctor today and he saw a polyp. It is not certain, but it might be cancerous." The news did not worry me that much. My mother's voice always had a victorious undertone. I always felt like my mom could fix or defeat anything. My response was serene. I wanted to know more. Why did she wait so long to address this medical issue? She always put her best on the outside. I would never suspect that she was sick.

"Don't worry," she said. "I will keep you informed when I know some-thing."

Mom called me after her ultrasound. She was not at all pleased with the young technician administrating the exam. The lab technician told her that he did not mean to disappoint her, but what he saw did not look good. He added that she had some type of cancer. On the phone my mother said, "Who is he to tell me I have cancer? How dare him. He is not a doctor!" I agreed with her. She was not willing to hear about the possibility of having cancer. Remember, my mother was able to fix or defeat anything.

This was the beginning of my family's life-changing experience. My mother was diagnosed with colorectal cancer. Many miles away from me, my mother underwent the most critical surgery of her life, and I could do nothing but pray and wait to hear the results. I called the hospital in New York several times that day and spoke to a nurse at the intensive care station. I was told she was stable and recovering. I thanked God and remained hopeful that things were going to turn out fine. My father eventually called to tell me that Mom was recovering well. He sounded very optimistic, and I felt well with the news that Mom had no complications despite her age.

My family and I went to New York City one month following the surgery. My mother had lost a lot of weight. She looked frail, but, emotionally, she was strong and in great spirits. She moved slower than usual. I made no spectacle of her appearance and embraced her. My dad did— a comment about how she was once again the dress size she was when they married. It was so different seeing her. Anything I could do to help my mother, I was more than willing to do. We attended her follow-up appointment with the surgeon. The wait was long. Several people sat in the waiting area, many of which were engrossed in their reading material. The office walls looked bland, and the receptionist greeted everyone with a warm smile. I sat next to my mom. My children sat half the time in my lap and the remainder sitting alone while flipping through the magazines on the table. My dad finally arrived after searching for a parking spot in New York's busy downtown area. My mother was finally called.

We were all invited to sit in the surgeon's office while he went over the surgery and where things would go from there. The news was hopeful, however, there was concern on the doctor's face. He told me that my mother was very fortunate. She was very sick. Her cancer was at stage three. My dad remembers the doctor saying that he had removed all that he could see. My father did not like the sound of that: "all that he could see." The doctor talked with encouragement, but his facial expression was bleak. He explained to us about the treatment that was ahead. The surgeon suggested that the treatment begin as soon as possible. It was a fight we all had to prepare for. After leaving the office, we stopped to pick up a few groceries. My mother said she was up for the task. I suggested she ride the electronic chair while I push the buggy. She refused.

"Mom, you should reserve your strength. Take it easy," I said.

"I am alright," she retorted.

I asked a young man working at the store if he could find us an electronic chair. I said subtly, "My mother isn't well enough to walk." The young man said, "I know." My mother said, "Excuse me? How does he know? I am fine. I don't need a chair!" she exclaimed. She insisted on walking the entire time we were there.

When I think back to that moment, I feel like I failed by making such an ordeal of her situation. The surgery was one thing to recover from. The treatment was another thing to get over. Now that she had endured the most critical surgery of her life, she was certainly dwelling on the idea of what to expect. I didn't know what emotional state she was in. She never needed anyone to do things for her. She was strong-willed. She was not going to ask for any help. I wish I had kept my big trap shut! I did not mean to cause her to feel incapable of caring for herself. Cancer is a whole lot for any person to really take in. A woman as independent, unselfish, and modest as my mom would not likely accept empathy from me, or anyone else for that matter. For my mom, it was business as usual. She picked up where she had left off. She resumed the responsibility of taking care of my oldest brother's children and household chores. She greatly appreciated the letter that my sister's friend had written to her about overcoming her personal battle with cancer. She shared the letter with me, and I remember the impression of courage she spoke with as she reread the letter. I would like to thank my sister's friend.

The day that my family and I planned to return to Atlanta, I did not want to leave. I remember telling my mother that if she needed me for anything, she could just call. We spoke for a long time while my husband packed the car. Mom looked so small. She was never overweight to begin with, yet, now, she looked underweight. Her clothes no longer fitted her. I said, again, "If you need me for anything just let me know." She said, "Take care of your husband and children." As she stood beside my dad she smiled and waved. I felt so sorrowful driving away and waving good-bye. With two young children in the back seat, the car ride out of the city was silent and uneventful.

Unnoticeable Change

Several months later, my mom had under gone several treatments of chemotherapy and radiation. I called her often and she would always re-assure me that she was well. Mother mentioned that she was gaining her weight back. She wanted to know how the children were doing and how everyone else was doing. She did not express to me what she was going through. While coping with her frequent treatments, she sounded really strong in spirit. It was my sister who shared with me the fact that Mom's fingertips were turning black and that she was beginning to experience hair loss. I had no idea that the treatments could be that severe. I had heard of the hair loss but never of one's fingertips and lips turning black.

Time and time again I asked my mother if there was anything I could do for her. "I will return home and help out," I would say. "No, no. You stay there and see about the children. I'll be alright," she said. Why did I listen? I did not realize, at the time, that I was speaking to my mother who was a new woman because of cancer. As much as I would have liked to continue to believe that my mother could beat the odds and fix anything, she was, in fact, a new woman. She was not the same person as before cancer invaded her life. She was the strong-willed, unstop-pable woman who raised me, but, at the same time, she was crippled by a disease that challenged her faith and pride. Sure, my mother was giving it all she had; she was trying to beat this thing. I didn't have to worry and she assured me. That was what I believed and longed to hear, but was this what she believed?

My dad recalled times that he would drive her to her appointments and she would say we are just wasting our time going back and forth to the treatment center. Dad said he would just say "No, no; we will go until you are all better." My mother was the strongest in the family; she was never doubtful. We were told by the surgeon to prepare ourselves for the fight ahead. I knew my mother was a strong Christian woman who believed that God could heal. She always displayed her best on the outside, even through turmoil and desperate times. There was no way she would lose this fight. The family could not see it or we did not want to believe it, but the truth was that she was changing.

It is hard to believe that cancer can happen to someone you love. It happened. It happened to my family, and my mother had no prior health issues that would have forewarned us, except for a fibroid tumor that she was told was not a threat. My dad later believed that was bad medical advice. We certainly did not foresee this happening. I had been so blinded by the perception of her being so close to perfect that I could not accept that life had changed. Mother was not the same anymore and neither were we.

As time moved on, I was less and less able to talk to my mother on the phone. When I called, she was either resting from the treatment or just not feeling well enough to talk. It was very unlike her to remain in bed during the day. I spoke briefly with my dad and sister who filled me in on my mother's appointments and how she was coping. Why did I not get on the first flight out of Atlanta? Why? Was I still under the notion that she was invincible? I worked in a Christian school and asked the teachers to pray for my mother. I believed that my mother would be delivered from her illness. My mother taught my siblings and me that by God's stripes we are healed. I knew God had the power to heal her, as stated in *Isaiah 5*. Mother said many times that all we could do was pray.

Time Flew By

The dream continued. There I was in a room full of gorgeous flowers. There were so many different hues blending together. It became more apparent that as the flowers continued to arrive in the room the image of her face grew more distraught. I felt a lot of love and warmth in the room. "Why do these flowers disappoint you? These flowers are from people who care about you," I said. Mother shook her head in dissatisfaction.

One late evening my siblings called me on a three-way call to discuss our mother's condition.

"I cannot believe it," my brother spoke surprisingly. "Mom could not walk. I carried her to the living room. This is scary, man! I mean, I have never seen Mom like this."

"What is happening?" I asked.

"Mom is in a lot of pain," my sister said. "I called the ambulance for her. I don't know. I am really worried."

I was informed that my mother could not hold herself up. My sister, brother, and I discussed talking with our parents about our mother's treatments and what to do should something go terribly wrong. It was time for a family talk. It was time for me to fly home. That was enough. I planned to go home and make arrangements for an elongated stay once I'd arrive in New York City. I was unable to talk with my mother for a few days and heard the news that she was in excruciating pain and couldn't walk. I wanted to crack up. Why? Why did I not leave when I was told she was too weak to receive my phone calls? Spring break was quickly approaching and school would be closed. I was definitely going to see my mother. While in the hospital, my dad said that Mom refused to eat. He would buy food from outside that was suitable for her diet but she refused it.

"She has got to eat! That is how she will regain her strength," he told me on the phone, flustered.

After days of not hearing her voice on the phone, I finally spoke to my mother in the hospital. She told me that a man was painting the frame of her hospital room door. What? I thought. She said it again; a man was painting the doorframe. Isn't that a health hazard to patients? I thought. How could the hospital allow this? Who would permit this while patients were in their rooms? In the background I heard a woman whining and muttering. I asked my mother what was going on. She said it was the patient in the bed beside her. She was extremely distressed and hurting. The woman was very loud. I asked my mother if she was okay with this going on. She told me the nurse had been in many times to console her neighbor, but she really didn't understand why she continued to wail. She said the nurse just pulled the curtain between them. I did not want to think about what was happening with anyone else but her. I suggested she request another room and shifted the conversation to Mother's condition.

"Are you eating, Mom?" I asked.

"I had a little this morning. I don't have an appetite," she replied.

I have heard that one of the side effects of chemo and radiation can be a loss of appetite. I recall how much weight my mother had lost after her surgery.

"Please try to eat," I said. "Do you have your Bible?"

"No," she replied. My sister was supposed to bring it to the hospital later that evening.

"We will keep praying for your healing," I said.

When I spoke to my father again, I asked about the interior painting going on around Mom's hospital room. He did not seem to be perturbed by it nor the fact that Mother's roommate was shrieking loudly. He did say that the upset patient had family that would visit from time to time.

My mother's health was dwindling. Only one week remained before my husband, children, and I planned to leave.

In New York City, the house my father and siblings knew was shaking apart. My sister made trips every day between work, school, and the hospital. My father spent many days by my mother's bedside, feeling helpless and worried. My brother had to find childcare for my nieces while Mom was hospitalized. My second brother and sister-in-law visited her when they could.

In Atlanta, my husband and I participated in Rick Warren's 40 Days of Community. During the final week of our Bible study group, I asked everyone to pray for my mother's healing. A kind neighbor gave me a book to give to my mother when I had arrived in New York. I wanted to be guided by God and to be filled with the Holy Spirit when I arrived at the hospital. I prayed that He would help me to minister to her. My in-laws would call the hospital to talk to her. I called several times during the last week before we were to leave Atlanta. Each time I spoke to my mother I would hear the patient in the hospital bed beside hers shouting and crying in distress in the background. What was happening? I thought. I could hardly hear my mother speak over her neighbor's cries.

"Does she have Alzheimer's?" I asked my mother.

My mother replied, but I didn't hear all that she said. I did hear her say the staff keeps the curtain closed. Dad said that Mom's condition remained about the same. She complained about high levels of pain, and the doctors increased her pain medication. The increase of dosage caused her to be incoherent, and my sister demanded that the doctors change it. According to my father, Mom tried to stay distracted by watching TV. I wondered what was going on. Why were the doctors not doing more? Her treatments were put off until she had regained some of her strength. The entire time she was hospitalized, she was not strong enough to get up from her bed. She had a catheter and used a bedpan to relieve herself.

I Didn't Hear a Thing

The last few days before we planned to leave Atlanta, I would call the hospital and sometimes not receive an answer. Other times my father would answer the phone. He sounded disheartened.

"How is she?" I asked.

"I don't know; she is unwilling to eat. She says her lower back continues to hurt," He replied. "The doctors are not certain themselves about what is going on."

"I will be there. I am leaving in three days," I told him. Dad gave the phone to my mother. I tried to sound cheerful.

"I will be there soon, Mom. Spring break begins Friday," I said.

She said okay.

"Hey," I said. "There is no more screaming. It is quiet there. How is the patient next to you?"

"Ooh," she paused. "She died."

"Oh my," I said.

"Yes," she said, "Poor thing. They have made her bed and opened the curtain."

I felt wretched. It was bizarre to hear this from my mother. For several days she laid ill in a hospital bed next to a woman we never knew, yet we had somehow became accustomed to her wailing and now we expressed sorrow that we would not know her or her cry again. The quiet was not welcomed. I did not like the news one bit and became more anxious to see her.

Tuesday afternoon I spoke with my mother. The conversation was very uncanny. I told her how I could not wait to see her. I said the children are excited about the trip, too. She said okay. I continued, "Well I hope that once we arrive in the city you will be out of there. I know you can't wait to get home." There was silence. I did not hear her respond. So, I said it again. "Mom, hopefully you will be out of the hospital when we arrive." Nothing but silence came across the phone. "Mom," I said and after a delay she answered, "Yes." I began to think that she was heavily medicated. I said, "Mom, are you okay? Is there someone there with you? You sound distracted." Her response was delayed.

"I am watching the teacher in the auditorium," she said.

I did not know how to respond. Was she hallucinating? "Mom, I will call back later alright?" She said alright. I held the phone to my ear until she hung up. I heard nothing but air on the other end. I placed the phone on the receiver after a while. I called my sister's cell phone numerous times until I was able to speak to her. She said she was going to the hospital after school and that she was disgusted with the doctor's treatment. So many doctors were involved with the situation and she wanted to contact one in particular. I talked to God that afternoon and asked Him to be there to take care of my mom.

Wednesday afternoon I called the hospital. Dad was very upset.

"Your momma is not doing well at all. I don't know what to do. She is complaining that she feels so much pain. Oh my Lord, she has pulled the IV out of her arm and blood is everywhere," he said

"Go get help! Go get the nurse and have her contact the doctor," I told him.

I wanted so much to talk to her. I knew she was in no mood to hold the phone. All I could think was, "Oh my, what is happening?" She continued to toss back and forth on her bed. Where was her nurse? I hung up and called back a few minutes later. The nurse was assisting in getting my mother to calm down. My dad said, "This is so unlike her." The change in her persona was no longer obscured from him. She was a new person.

"She can't get comfortable. The nurse said she has placed a call to her doctor," my father said in an upset voice. I told my dad to attend to her and that I would call back later. My heart became heavy. Many miles away, what could I do? I could do the very thing she taught me to do. I looked around my house, and in the center of the floor I fell to my knees. Alone in my living room I cried out to God. I cried and prayed. I prayed long and hard asking God to deliver my mother from the pain she was enduring and for her healing. I asked in Jesus' name. I continued to sob while the children were not around. I sat, calling on God to comfort my mom. In just two more days I would be there. I would bring scripture to recite and believed God would heal her.

About three hours later I called the hospital. My dad's voice seemed invigorated.

"How is she?" I asked.

"Oh! She got up!" I could hear the smile on his face. "She walked to the bathroom. I cannot believe it," he said. "I tried to hold on to her arm, but she suddenly wanted to get up."

Dad's voice was full of amazement and wonder.

"Yes, wow. She walked to the bathroom. No assistance at all, I tell you."

I was smiling on the phone as I was taking in all that had just transpired in the past four hours.

"Thank you, Lord," I said. I told my dad how I had just prayed for her.

"Yes. Really," he replied.

Hope was alive. I said I would call back and hung up the phone. I thanked God. He heard my prayers. I spent the rest of the evening telling my husband about the events that had happened. I called my mother's sister to tell her what had transpired. This was encouraging news for everyone.

It was springtime and my allergies were not causing me a problem. However, I did not rest easy on that night. I tried everything I could to fall asleep. After midnight, I wandered downstairs and felt a familiar sensation come over me. It lasted for a few seconds and it stopped. I had felt this before and could not understand why it was happening again. I got a drink of water and sat up for a few more hours until I was finally able to get some rest.

Tomorrow Never Ends

That morning was typical. I scrambled to get the children and myself ready for school. Just as we were all packed and set to get into the car, my phone rang. I looked at the phone and then answered. It was my sister. With much dismay in her voice, she said, "Mom died!" My heart felt like it was stomping in my chest. I heard myself say, "What!"

She repeated, "Mom has died!"

"Oh. Oh my. No! No! Mom has died," I repeated. My husband took the phone, and I ran around the house crying, "No! No! No! I dialed my mother's sister and spoke with distress and disbelief. "Mom has died," I said.

"I heard," she answered. Her voice was low and somber. "You are going to have to calm yourself down or you will upset the children," she said. "I am on the phone with your dad and sister, and I will call you back."

My husband called out of work and we actually drove the children to school. I told my administrators what had happened. I was excused from my job. My husband drove the car back home. I didn't want to believe this day was happening. Just like the car ride out of New York City, the car ride home was silent and uneventful.

On that day, life was happening and my mother was no longer around. Was this real? I kept looking sharply at my surroundings to see if life was happening around me, at the clear blue sky, the green tree limbs blowing in the wind, the cars passing by. I could feel it, I could see it and, yet, I could not hear a thing. Every authentic sound was drowned out. The constant wailing of my mother's bunkmate returned, only it was not the distressed hospital patient beside her any longer; it was me. Internally, I was then, and I still am, screaming. I am screaming because each new day does not change the fact that she is no longer a part of it. This fact does not change, so tomorrow never ends. I scream because cancer happened. It happened to my family. I better understand the shrieking that goes on inside.

I can now hear my mother's silent responses on the phone. My dad said she tried to stay distracted by watching TV. She did not hear it. The reason she was not overwhelmed by her neighbor's cries was simply because she was screaming internally. She was putting up the best fight she could. Those affected by cancer scream to find a better explanation, a better cure, a better way out of this mess happening to them. I am still putting up a fight. God knows our endings before our beginnings. I have learned that things work out according to His will and purpose. It was not His will that cancer prevail over my mother. God's will was that, through my mother, He would receive the glory. Her life was not in vain. I now comprehend the dream I had weeks prior to my mother's transition. I didn't hear her response; however, her demeanor spoke loud and clear.

There I was in a room full of gorgeous flowers. There were so many different hues blending together. It became more apparent that as the flowers continued to arrive in the room, the image of her face grew more distraught. I felt a lot of love and warmth in the room. "Why do these flowers disappoint you? These flowers are from people who care about you," I said. Mother shook her head in dissatisfaction. The vision faded away.

I Remember
by Melissa Saunders

I remember like it was yesterday when I last saw my grandmommy. I remember great things about her. I remember the delicious breakfast she made for us, the cookies she gave us, and more. I remember her smiling at me. My little brother and I would smile back at her. I did not understand what was happening. I did not know she was very sick with a disease called cancer. We stayed in an apartment. Around the apartment was a lot of fancy equipment. Unknown to me, the equipment was for Grandma's health. After a few days in New York we returned to Atlanta. Many months later, when I was five, my mom got the call that Grandma had died. My mom cried and cried. When she drove us to school, I could tell she was sad. I was too. I think my brother was sad. At the funeral I cried. My mother shed tears like a big whale. It was a sad time for my family.

Recently, I learned some more things about Grandmommy. In third grade I had to write a report on someone in my family who had cancer. I asked my mother if anyone in our family had cancer. She answered, "Yes, your grandmommy. She died from cancer." I found out it was colon cancer. I wrote my report about Grandmommy's good days and her not-so-good days. I participated in a relay race and wore a blue ribbon. When I ran, I wore a special shirt with a blue ribbon on it. I ran that race. I did not finish first, but I ran for my grandmommy. I ran for her. I love her and will never forget her. Her memory will stay in my heart. I know I will see her again in a wonderful place, and it is called Heaven.